Scientific Writing
Handbook

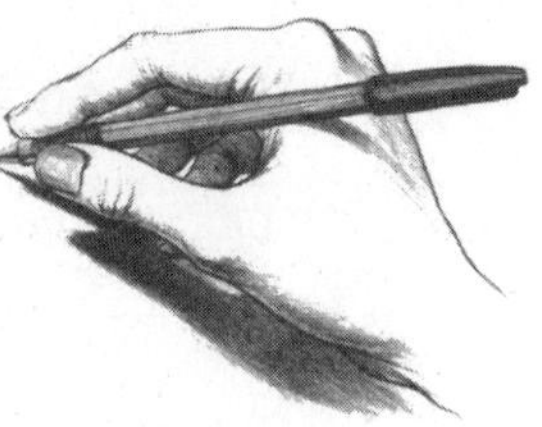

Scientific Writing Handbook

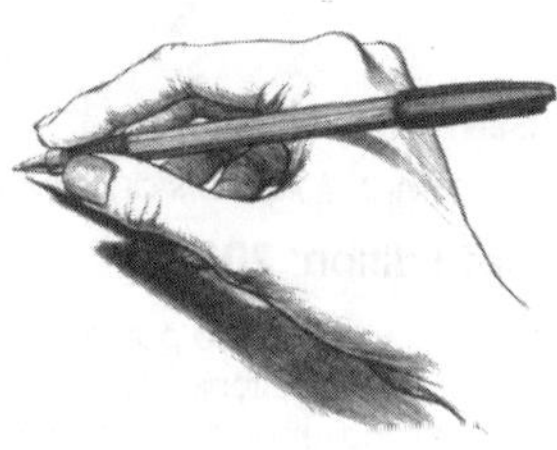

S Kalpana
MSc (Faculty of Medicine) MBA (HA) PhD (Immunology)
Research Officer
Department of Epidemiology
The Tamil Nadu Dr MGR Medical University
Guindy, Chennai, Tamil Nadu

K Kanimozhi
BDS MSc (Epidemiology)
Dental Consultant and Epidemiologist
Editorial Board Member for International and
National Medical and Dental Journals

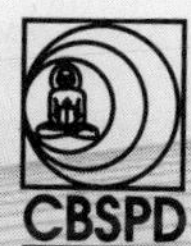

CBSPD

CBS Publishers & Distributors Pvt Ltd

New Delhi • Bengaluru • Chennai • Kochi • Kolkata • Lucknow • Mumbai
Hyderabad • Jharkhand • Nagpur • Patna • Pune • Uttarakhand

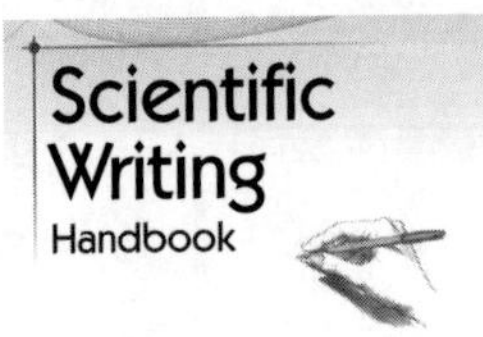

Scientific Writing
Handbook

ISBN: 978-93-5466-789-3

Copyright © Authors and Publisher

First Edition: 2025

Published by **Satish Kumar Jain** and produced by **Varun Jain** for

CBS Publishers & Distributors Pvt Ltd

4819/XI Prahlad Street, 24 Ansari Road, Daryaganj, New Delhi 110 002, India
Ph: 011-23289259, 23266838   Website: www.cbspd.com
                                    e-mail: delhi@cbspd.com

Corporate Office: 204 FIE, Industrial Area, Patparganj, Delhi 110 092, India
Ph: 011-4934 4934   Fax: 011-4934 4935   e-mail: publishing@cbspd.com; publicity@cbspd.com

Branches

- **Bengaluru:** Seema House 2975, 17th Cross, K.R. Road, Banasankari 2nd Stage, Bengaluru 560 070, Karnataka, India
  Ph: +91-80-26771678/79   Fax: +91-80-26771680   e-mail: bangalore@cbspd.com
- **Chennai:** 7, Subbaraya Street, Shenoy Nagar, Chennai 600 030, Tamil Nadu, India
  Ph: +91-44-26680620, 26681266   Fax: +91-44-42032115   e-mail: chennai@cbspd.com
- **Kochi:** 42/1325, 1326, Power House Road, Opposite KSEB, Power House, Ernakulum, Kochi-682 018, Kerala, India
  Ph: +91-484-4059061–67   Fax: +91-484-4059065   e-mail: kochi@cbspd.com
- **Kolkata:** 147, C/o Hind Ceramics Compound,, 1st Floor, Nilgunj Road, Belghoria, Kolkata-700 056, West Bengal, India
  Ph: +91-33-25633055/56   e-mail: kolkata@cbspd.com
- **Lucknow:** Basement, Khushnuma Complex, 7-Meerabai Marg (behind Jawahar Bhawan), Lucknow-226 001, Uttar Pradesh, India.
  Ph: +91-522-4000032   e-mail: tiwari.lucknow@cbspd.com
- **Mumbai:** PWD Shed, Gala No. 25/26, Ramchandra Bhatt Marg, Next to JJ Hospital, Gate No. 2, Opp Union Bank of India, Noorbaug, Mumbai-400009, Maharashtra, India.
  Ph: +91-22-66661880, 66661889   e-mail: mumbai@cbspd.com

Representatives

• **Hyderabad**	0-9885175004	• **Jharkhand**	0-9811541605	• **Nagpur**	0-8692091830
• **Patna**	0-9334159340	• **Pune**	0-9664372571	• **Uttarakhand**	0-9716462459

Printed at: Glorious Printer, Jhilmil Industrial Area, Delhi, India

to

---

our brothers,
Mr S Stalin and Mr S Nepolian

Foreword

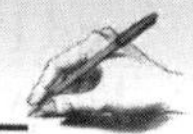

I am honoured to introduce the *Scientific Writing Handbook,* written by Dr S Kalpana and Dr K Kanimozhi. This handbook serves as a guiding light, illuminating the path for readers to become adept and influential communicators within the intricate realm of research. It provides a roadmap to navigate the complexities of scholarly communication, empowering novices to confidently present their research findings as manuscripts, while offering seasoned scholars a platform to refine their skills.

Tailored to a diverse audience, this book caters to undergraduate and postgraduate students and PhD aspirants from diverse academic backgrounds, functioning as a dependable companion, simplifying the journey through the scientific landscape. Covering essential topics such as manuscript structuring, formatting, ethical considerations, plagiarism, research integrity, editing, peer review, as well as the nuances of crafting systematic reviews and meta-analyses, significance of indexed journals and the role of impact factors, this handbook ensures readers attain a holistic grasp of scholarly writing. It undoubtedly attests to the unwavering dedication and expertise of its authors in the realm of research and scholarly communication.

Dr S Kalpana, a dedicated researcher at The Tamil Nadu Dr MGR Medical University's Department of Epidemiology, Chennai, has over 25 years of experience in publishing and academic mentorship. Her legacy shines in this guide, enriched by her numerous international and national journal articles. As a reviewer for esteemed journals, she upholds high academic standards, reflecting her commitment to advancing knowledge. Dr K Kanimozhi brings a decade's worth of publishing expertise. Her role as a reviewer for reputable international and national journals, along with memberships on editorial boards, showcases her dedication to enhancing scholarly work's quality. My acquaintance with her dates back to her role as a Consultant under the Department of Health and Family Welfare for the National Health Mission (NHM), Government of Tamil Nadu. Her unwavering dedication to healthcare and research remains commendable. Dr Krishna

Prasanth is a epidemiologist, working in Balaji Medical College and Hospital. He is a public health person who has vast research knowledge and published many research papers in national and international journals has also helped in drafting some contents of this book. This handbook is a testment to the profound expertise of both authors in their respective fields, reflecting their relentless pursuit of research excellence and commitment to nurturing future scholars. The remarkable diligence invested in creating this guide is evident.

As readers delve into its contents, they will discover a treasure trove of knowledge, expert insights, and practical techniques. This resource will not only refine their writing skills but also amplify their impact within the academic community. This handbook underscores the authors' commitment and has the power to transform how scholars approach communicating scientific ideas through their academic journey.

I extend my best wishe to the readers of this book, encouraging them to embrace the tools and wisdom presented within. May this guide empower them to become exceptional researchers, leaving an indelible mark on the scientific world through their scholarly works.

Dr TS Selvavinayagam
MD DPH DNB (Health and Hospital Administration)
Director
Public Health and Preventive Medicine
Department of Health and Family Welfare
Government of Tamil Nadu, India

Foreword 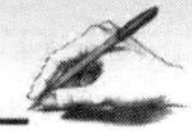

It is my distinct privilege to introduce the *Scientific Writing Handbook* authored by Dr S Kalpana and Dr K Kanimozhi. Contained within these pages is evidence of their profound expertise, serving as a testament to their unwavering dedication to achieving research excellence and their significant impact on shaping the forthcoming generation of scholars. Dr S Kalpana's enduring legacy as a dedicated research officer in the Department of Epidemiology at The Tamil Nadu Dr MGR Medical University, radiates through every page of this handbook. With an illustrious career spanning over 25 years in publishing her substantial collection of international and national journal articles attests to her remarkable contributions to the research landscape. Beyond her impressive academic accomplishments, her role as a revered journal reviewer portrays her unwavering commitment to upholding scholarly standards. Notable, her role as a guide for numerous students further exemplifies her profound influence on shaping the next generation of scholars.

The handbook stands as a testimony to her unwavering journey of advancing the frontiers of knowledge. Dr K Kanimozhi brings a decade's worth of valuable experience in the publishing domain. Her role as a dedicated reviewer for the reputed Elsevier CEGH journal, coupled with her involvement on other national and international editorial boards as renowned editorial board member, showcases her dedication to elevating the quality of scholary work. Her passion for continuous learning is evident through her active participation in diverse courses, ranging from research methology to the refined art of journal reviewing. Also, the contributions of few content by Dr Krishna Prasanth who is an epidemiologist, working in the Balaji Medical College and Hospital, is also remarkable. He has vast research knowledge and has published many research papers in national and international journals.

This handbook goes beyond being a mere complication of knowledge. It embodies the authors' relentless pursuit of research excellence and their sincere endeavour to pave the way for the next generation of scholars. The diligence they have poured into creating this comprehensive guide is nothing short of remarkable. As you, dear readers, immerse yourselves in its pages, you will unrearth a treasure of knowledge and expert guidance. Thses resources are poised to not only refine your writing skills but also amplify your contributions within the academic community.

This handbook, a testament to the authors' dedication, has the potential to reshape the very approach scholars take at each juncture of their journey in conveying scientific ideas. In your hands, you hold more than a guide; you hold the collective wisdom of researchers who have not only navigated the intricate landscapes of scientific communication but have also enriched them.

It is my sincere belief that this handbook will inspire and empower you to become exceptional researchers, leaving an indelible mark on the scientific world through your scholarly endeavours.

01/09/23

Dr (Prof) Shally Awasthi
Head, Department of Pediatrics
and Medical Education
Dean
Research and Development
King George's Medical University
Lucknow, UP, India

Preface

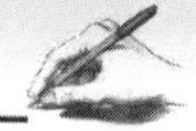

Embarking on the path of scientific research is both thrilling and daunting. This comprehensive handbook delves into the intricacies of scholarly publication, offering a guiding light for researchers navigating the complexities of the academic world by providing invaluable insights and practical advice distilled from years of our collective experience in scientific writing. From grasping the nuances of research publication to mastering the structure of a manuscript, each section is carefully curated. Noteworthy features of this book include further readings, suggestions as well as chapter summaries, which highlight key concepts for enhanced understanding. Delving into crafting impactful titles, abstracts, and keywords, this book also provides guidance on composing each section of a manuscript, from introduction to discussion and conclusion, guiding researchers through the meticulous process of crafting each section with precision and clarity. Additionally, vital topics such as authorship, plagiarism, copyright, research ethics, and the peer review process are addressed. With a dedicated section on manuscript formatting, this book equips researchers at all levels with the necessary tools for effective communication of their work. Whether embarking on a first publication journey or refining writing skills as a seasoned academic, this handbook empowers researchers to navigate the intricate landscape of scientific writing with confidence. This comprehensive guide, sets the stage for an enriching and rewarding journey in the realm of scientific research and publication.

We sincerely thank to Dr B Krishna Prasanth for his meticulous proofreading work, which has greatly enriched the quality of this handbook.

S Kalpana
K Kanimozhi

Acknowledgements

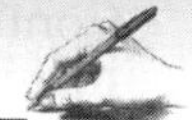

We embark on this noble endeavor with profound gratitude, as the benevolent guidance of the Almighty has graciously illuminated our path, leading us to fruition. We owe an immense debt of gratitude to both of our families, whose boundless love, support, and understanding have served as unwavering pillars of strength. Their steadfast belief in our capabilities has propelled us forward with determination to see this project through to completion.

We are deeply honored and privileged to have esteemed dignitaries such as Dr TS Selvavinayagam, Director of Public Health, Government of Tamil Nadu, and Dr Shally Awasthi, Head, Department of Pediatrics and Dean, Research and Development, King George's Medical University, Uttar Pradesh, grace this handbook with their insightful forewords. Their expertise and esteemed perspectives have added immense credibility and depth to our work, laying a robust foundation for its reception and impact.

Furthermore, we extend our heartfelt gratitude to Dr K Narayanasamy, Vice Chancellor, The Tamil Nadu Dr MGR Medical University, Chennai, for his unwavering support and encouragement. His exemplary leadership and guidance have been invaluable in navigating the challenges and realizing the vision of this handbook.

We are greatly indebted to Dr Manjula Datta, our mentor, for her profound knowledge and dedication to excellence, which has greatly enriched the writing of this book. Her mentorship has not only enhanced the quality of the content but has also fostered our growth as writers and scholars.

We would like to thank Dr G Srinivas, Professor and Head, Department of Epidemiology, The Tamil Nadu Dr MGR Medical University, Chennai, for his motivation and constant support to complete this handbook.

We are deeply grateful to Dr Parameswari Srijayanth, Controller of Examination, Dr MGR Educational and Research Institute, Maduravoyal, Chennai, for her wisdom and unwavering belief in our abilities.

Additionally, our sincere appreciation goes to Dr B Krishna Prasanth, Associate Professor, Sree Balaji Medical College, Chennai, for his meticulous proof reading efforts, which have elevated the clarity, coherence, and overall quality of our work.

We reserve our utmost gratitude to CBS Publishers & Distributor notably Mr YN Arjuna and Ms Jassi, whose support has been pivotal from the inception of this handbook as a mere draft to its tangible presence. Their unwavering assistance has guided us at every phase of this transformative journey. Our heartfelt appreciation for their invaluable guidance and encouragement throughout this endeavor.

To all those who have contributed, seen and unseen, we express our gratitude. It is through the collective efforts that we have been able to bring this project to fruition, and for that, we are truly thankful.

Lastly, we extend our gratitude to you, our beloved readers, for taking the time to read our book and improve your knowledge of scientific writing.

Our sincere best wishes extend to all researchers as we fervently hope for their triumph and fulfillment in their scholarly pursuits.

S Kalpana
K Kanimozhi

Contents

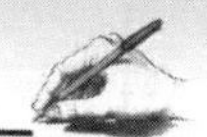

Abbreviations

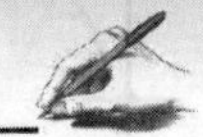

JIF: Journal Impact Factor

SNIP: Scopus's source Normalised Index per Paper

IMRaD: Introduction, Materials and Methods, Results and Discussion

PICO: Population, Intervention, Comparison and Outcome

SEO: Search Engine Optimisation

PRISMA: Preferred Reporting Items for Systematic reviews and Meta Analysis.

RCT: Randomised Control Trial

CONSORT: COnsolidated Standards Of Reporting Trials

ICMJE: International Committee of Medical Journal Editors

IAIP: Institutional Academy Integrity Panel

IRB: Institutional Review Board

MeSH: Medical Subject Headings

GIGO: Garbage In and Garbage Out

ISSN: International Standard Serial Number

PMC: PubMed Central

NLM: National Library of Medicine

SCIE: Science Citation Index Expanded

ESCI: Emerging Sources Citation Index

H index: Hirsch index

Art of Research Publication 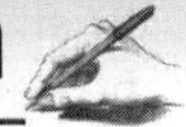

*"There are two things people want more than money.
Recognition and Praise."*

—Mark Kay Ash

Introduction

In the realm of academia, the quantity and quality of research articles that a researcher or faculty produces within a given year holds a significant place in various facets of their professional journey. Academic institutions routinely prioritize the assessment of a researcher's publication history when making pivotal decisions, right from the recruitment of new faculty members to the evaluation of existing ones and also in the determination of promotions. Scholarly publications not only play a critical role in gauging the effectiveness and contributions of faculty members but also serve as a key factor in their eligibility for research fellowships, prestigious awards, and research grants. Furthermore, the attainment of tenure, which provides a sense of job security and signals a long-term commitment to the academic institution, often hinges on the strength of a researcher's publication record. Beyond the quantity of publications, the quality, influence and relevance of the research are of paramount importance. These factors contribute significantly to a researcher's academic reputation and help them maintain their position within their specific field. In essence, a scholar's publication record acts as a comprehensive metric of their intellectual contributions and their capability to advance their career within the academic sphere.

Having a research project published in a peer-reviewed publication has advantages for both the researcher and the researcher's host institution. The reason for this is that there is a lot of competition for jobs in the field. Indeed, even before students complete their doctoral degrees, there is pressure to start publishing their work. Many postgraduate students nowadays want to publish their work while they are still pursuing their degrees to improve their prospects of obtaining placement after graduation. This book is meant to serve as a guide for students (undergraduate, postgraduate and PhD) of medical, paramedical, and allied health sciences, who are unsure, how to publish their journal papers. Additionally, students are encouraged to collaborate with their academic supervisors, who possess valuable expertise and insights into the publication process specific to their respective fields of study.

Medical science is fully reliant on scientific facts being reported in scientific journals, newspapers, and magazines. According to their needs, each speciality in medical science has its journals and innovative ways of publication. Researchers benefit from publishing several types of scientific papers from a variety of perspectives. New researchers are more likely to publish original research to progress their careers, whereas specialists are more likely to use other sorts of publications to obtain their authorial voice in influencing a larger audience.

Publication is the means through which any study, along with its scientific and practical contributions, is conveyed to peers within its respective field. This helps to develop knowledge and its application by informing scientific researchers and practitioners with similar interests about new knowledge in their sector. Higher-quality journals are more challenging to publish in, but they demonstrate competence in a topic and the capacity to conduct scientifically sound research. It also shows the academic standing of the institution that hosted the publication. Scientific data is available to submissions from a wide range of topics in the natural, clinical, and social sciences, including descriptions and analysis of huge and small data, from major consortiums, single labs, and individuals. Publishing with scientific data provides citable, peer-reviewed credit for collected datasets. Even after the hard effort that produced publishable results, writing a manuscript, and having it published in a peer-reviewed journal is difficult. So, what motivates people to engage in such behaviour? What drives the authors to complete the writing process and then submit their work for peer review? Altruism and self-interest are the two types of motivations, and most authors have a mix of both.

In the present scientific world, peer-reviewed science journals serve as the predominant platform for altruistically sharing and preserving scientific breakthroughs. Science evolves and progresses remarkably as a collective reservoir of knowledge that is perpetually tested, refined, and expanded upon. For many scientists, their primary motivation for entering the field lies in their deep-seated desire to advance their respective domains for the betterment of society. They view publishing in reputable journals as a straightforward and altruistic means to make this valuable contribution, which in turn serves as a powerful source of motivation in their pursuit of scientific excellence.

Self-interest in writing and publishing a paper can also provide concrete rewards to an author, offering a self-interested reason for doing so. Publishing is frequently accompanied by direct or indirect monetary rewards, and it may be essential for career advancement. In academia, the well-known "Publish or Perish" paradigm adds a proverbial stick to the incentive of promotion. Even if they do not have these evident professional motives, practically everyone wants to be recognized for their work. As everyone feels, "I am well aware that the benefit of peer recognition motivates me much."

A literature search should always be the first step in any new research effort. The purpose of the search is to assess the current state of our collective knowledge on a topic before beginning a quest to add to it. Since, science revolves around the processes of verifying, challenging, or generating novel information, making a strong grasp of the existing knowledge is a fundamental prerequisite for the five purposes of citations. It is important to remember that a literature search is not about discovering relevant papers; it is about reading them thoroughly. Regrettably, literature searches are rarely carried out as thoroughly as they should be. Here are some pointers to help you enhance your literature searches:

- The most promising papers to read are the frequently cited articles which are relevant to your field of research.
- Also, look for literature beyond your discipline
- Although keeping track of prior publications as reference is a good beginning, it is essential to recognize that no one can fully grasp the entire breadth of literature, even within the most specialized subject areas. Thus, it is unwise to depend solely on one's memory.
- Look for recent papers on the subject as you finish your manuscript.

Other academicians may be working on similar themes and have published papers that you should study to ensure that your article contains the most up-to-date information in the field. When beginning a literature search, a challenging question often arises: how do you know when to stop? There will always be critical documents that you are unable to locate. This is how modern science works. It is a matter of judgment and experience to know when to stop the literature search and start working on a new project. If so, the research should be planned and executed with publication in mind. As discussed throughout this manual, one of the critical requirements of a science paper is to document the work in sufficient aspect so that the reader can follow the analysis presented and validate the conclusions drawn. Furthermore, authors of a published work must be enthusiastic to defend their work against criticism, so they should always keep the raw data and crucial details about the experimental technique on hand for later evaluation. First and foremost, these objectives necessitate meticulous laboratory record-keeping. The "lab notebook" has traditionally performed this purpose, albeit it is now more typically a virtual notebook containing well-organized digital information. Knowing what information, you will need from these records to write a paper might help you keep track of your records. For instance, if you check the standards for what is necessary in a method section of a paper, you will be aware of the record-keeping needs for authoring the method section easily. Before your data is published as an article, raw data is frequently altered, reformatted, filtered, summarised, and graphed. At each of these steps, it virtually always required that the data be archived. You do not want to be in a situation where the graph's "image" is the only thing that remains of the original data when you publish it.

What and where to publish?

There are many forums to present your research work, as depicted in Fig. 1, and they have been briefed below:

* **Articles**—a unique, brief written item that may or may not include photographs and is generally focused on current topics.
* **Books**—usually a large amount of information published all at once. But this requires a considerable deal of effort from both the author and the publisher as it is voluminous.
* **Newspapers**—in most cases, a daily publication of social, political, and lifestyle events.
* **Websites**—a digital item made up of multiple pages created by someone with technical skills or even your technical skills can be utilized by someone else, which would also have monetary benefits.
* **Conference papers**—a written version of a presentation given at a professional or research conference. In this case, the authors are usually working professionals or academicians in their respective fields.
* **Documentaries**—a production, such as a film or television programme, that presents political, social, or historical subject matter in a factual and informative manner, frequently consisting of genuine news footage or interviews with narrators.
* **Magazines/Journals**—published regularly, they contain many articles that are edited and selected and are relevant to some broad or specific professional research interest.
* **Blogs**—a frequently updated website that does not require substantial technical knowledge and can be created by almost anyone for no expense other than the time, they invest to create the content. Usually identified by postings with the date on which they were written.

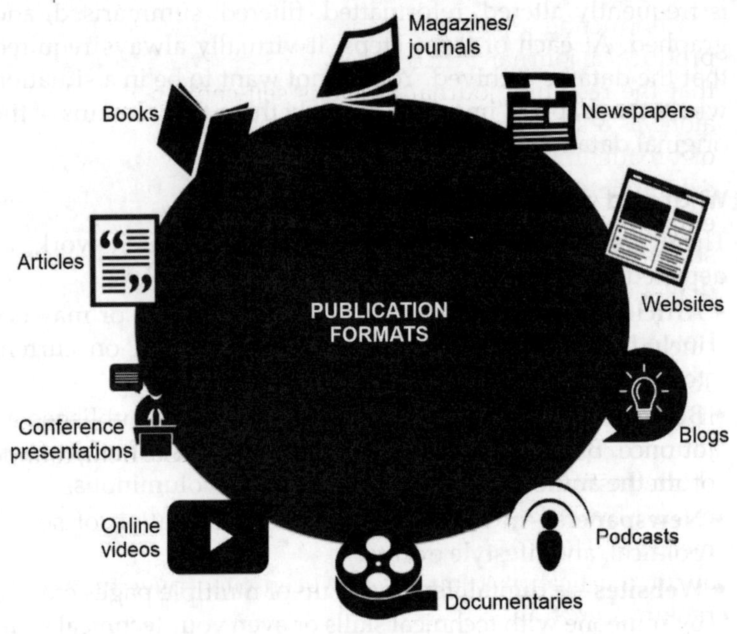

Fig. 1: Publication formats

The first choice a researcher must make is whether to convert one particular chapter from his or her thesis into a journal article or to compose the whole thesis as a separate journal. Both options have pros and cons. It is critical to make the right choice and ensure that the material is appropriate when using a chapter (or multiple chapters) from a thesis as the foundation for a journal article. A journal article must be a self-contained piece of study; it cannot refer to information from other portions of the thesis that are not included in the journal article. The journal article should establish a specific topic, include unique scholarly research on that topic, and be independent. Of course, one advantage of transforming a thesis chapter into a journal article rather than starting a new research project is that the researcher will not be adding to his or her workload at a time when they are already overburdened. Another benefit is that if a student can successfully publish a piece of their thesis in a peer-reviewed journal during their degree, it is a good sign that the thesis will be accepted by examiners.

Conducting a separate and smaller research project to produce a journal article offers the advantage of ensuring that the resulting journal article is self-contained and stands alone as a separate piece of work. It also provides the benefit of broadening your knowledge and competence, as well as exhibiting the skills that many employers seek from their employees. The negative is that it will necessitate additional study before an article can be published, which can be time demanding.

How to select a journal?

To determine a journal's standing or relative prominence in it is subject, several journal ranking systems are utilized. The Journal Impact Factor (JIF), created by Eugene Garfield, founder of the Institute for Scientific Information, which is currently owned by Thomson Reuters, is one of the most well-known methods. The JIF is a metric that measures how frequently an average article in a journal has been cited over time. Other rankings, such as SNIP (Scopus's Source Normalized Index per Paper) and the Google Scholar Index, are also used. The value of a researcher, who is often a faculty member, PhD student, or research fellow at an academic institution, can be measured using a journal's ranking.

Before you start writing your paper, think about in which publication you would like to see it published. This is because each magazine has its own set of formatting, style, and citation rules. To save time, draft your journal article first according to the rules of the journal where you want to publish it.

When selecting the journal or journals in which you want to be published, there are several criteria to consider. You should make a list of appropriate periodicals in order of choice. To begin, look for a list of all journals in your field of study on the internet or through your university's library website.

While journal quality and reputation are important, you may not want to aim for the highest-quality or highest-ranked journal in your field for your first publication, as this may increase the chances of your article being rejected. Make a list of five to ten journals in which you would like your article to be published and most importantly, approach them one at a time.

How to start writing?

Once you have chosen the journal to which you will submit your article, go to the journal's website to learn more about the format, style, and language criteria. You must follow the journal's specific and individual criteria exactly. These rules will also tell you how long your post should be in general, with minimum and maximum lengths being provided. Check whether the article is written in British/Australian or American English (as per the guidelines of the journal), as well as which referencing style to use and how to structure it.

If you have converted a chapter of your thesis into a journal article, stick to the journal's guidelines because your thesis follows a different pattern.

Before submission

First, make sure that you follow all the publisher's guidelines properly when writing your article. Second, look up information about the journal's submission process on its website. It is critical, once again, that you adhere to the journal's specific and unique standards. Some journals only accept electronic submissions, while others allow either or both formats. Read the journal's criteria when submitting your first article. It is critical to submit journal papers to only one journal at a time when submitting them for consideration. If an article is being considered for publication elsewhere, almost all journals will decline to consider it for publication. Most journals will ask you to declare that your work is not currently under review elsewhere as part of the official submission procedure.

After submission

The peer review method acts as a quality assurance system. Before an article may be approved for publication, it is subjected to peer review by a board of experts in the field who examine it for relevance, and quality, and confirm if the submitted work aligns with the scientific standards as well as the editorial standards of the respective journal. To assist, in removing prejudice, peer review is done blind (that is, neither the reviewer nor the author knows the identity of each other). The peer review process is normally coordinated by the journal's editor.

The peer-reviewing procedure can take a long time. The formal verdict of the journal can take anything from 6 weeks to 6 months to arrive. A two-stage review method is used by several periodicals. The paper will first be reviewed by one of the journal's editors to see if it is worthy of peer review. If your article passes the first review, it will be sent to one or more anonymous peer reviewers for a second opinion (academicians who are experts in the field upon which you have written). After what may seem like an eternity, you will receive an email or a letter from the journal informing you of their response to the work that you have submitted. The decision is frequently accompanied by reports or comments from the reviewers. If your manuscript has been denied for publication, you must request the reviewers' reports or comments since it may contain essential information that you can utilize to enhance your manuscript before submitting it to another academic journal.

It is uncommon for a first-time author's first journal paper to be accepted for publication by the first journal to which it is submitted. Congratulations if this happens to you! However, do not be discouraged if it does not. Rejection is an inevitable aspect of the publication process, and every author has been turned down at some point. If your article is rejected, if at all possible, use the reviewer's remarks to enhance it. After that, you will need to get your article ready to be sent to the next journal on your list.

Only if it is subject to revision, will it be accepted. Anything other than "reject" is a positive assessment, according to Ms Neal-Barnett. These are some of them:

- **Accept:** "Which virtually nobody understands"
- **Accept with a stipulation:** "Just make a few minor adjustments."
- **Revise and resubmit:** "They are still interested in you!". So, according to the reviewers' comments, revise your article and resubmit it.
- **Reject and resubmit:** "They still want the paper!" even if it is not as good as revise and resubmit.

Every criticism should be viewed as a good recommendation for something you could better explain. Put the review aside once you have read it the first time. Return to it later, carefully reviewing the document to determine whether the critiques were valid and how you may respond to them. Reviewers frequently make remarks that are off-target as a result of misinterpreting some parts of your paper. If this is the case, then do not let it bother you; simply rewrite that section of your paper more explicitly so that the same misunderstanding does not occur again. It is aggravating to have a paper rejected due to a miscommunication, but it is something you can correct. On the other hand, complaints about the paper is content may necessitate more extensive adjustments, such as reconsidering your ideas and conducting further testing. If your paper is turned down, do not give up! Take the feedback seriously and try to modify the article in response to the reviewer's suggestions. "Keep in mind that if you want to obtain a lot of publications, you will have to get a lot of rejections."

Further suggestions:
1. Websites for reviewing the literature:
    - Pubmed
    - Scopus
    - Embase
    - Web of science
    - Wizdom.ai
    - Semantic scholar
    - Google scholar
    - Microsoft academic search
    - Scinapse
    - Proquest
    - EBSCO
2. Citation-based article identifiers (to identify the most cited relevant articles):
    - Societies
    - Scite.ai
    - Researcher app
    - Microsoft academic

3. Literature analysis:
   - Microsoft academic
   - Semantic
   - Scopus
   - Web of science
   - Scinapase.io
   - Scholarly
   - Paper digest
   - Unpay wall

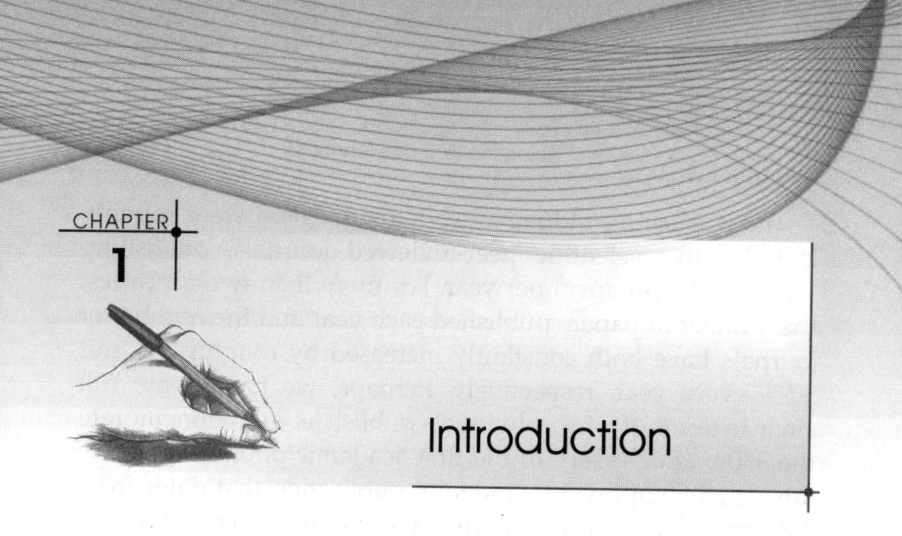

Introduction

"Academic success depends on research and publications."

—Philip Zimbardo

The scientific writing process can be daunting and is frequently postponed as the "final step" in the scientific process, resulting in haphazard attempts to put scientific ideas and results on paper. Scientific investigations are rigorous and interesting efforts, but they must be communicated to others to make an influence. A research paper is an attempt to communicate with others about the specific data that has been acquired as a resultant of your study and what you think those data represent in the context of your research. The "rules" for writing a scientific paper are strict and distinct from those for writing an English theme or a library research article. The paper requires adequate use of the English language for clear communication, and this will be taken into account when evaluating your study reports. Scientific papers must be written with clarity and be simple so that readers with similar backgrounds may quickly grasp what you have done and how you did it if they want to replicate or extend your work. You can presume that your audience will be readers with similar understanding when writing articles for your field of specialization. Scientific writing, on the other hand, should begin far before the first plan is written. Researching how your work fits within the current literature, constructing an engaging plot, and determining how best you can adapt your message to an intended audience are all essential components of successful writing.

The publishing industry is booming. There were roughly 28,100 active scientific peer-reviewed journals, publishing 1.8–1.9 million papers per year. For more than two centuries, the number of papers published each year and the number of journals have both constantly increased by roughly 3% and 3.5% every year, respectively. Perhaps, we have come full circle in terms of why individuals publish as we commemorate the 350th anniversary of the first academic publication. Why are we still employing a mode of publication that dates from 1665 in this age of the internet and social media? What is a journal in the twenty-first century, and what role does it play? Surprisingly, since its inception 350 years ago, the academic journal has remained unchanged.

Journals are important in academic life for more reasons than just providing a means of communication and a permanent record. Most research culminates in journal papers, and a researcher's productivity and performance are measured in large part by the number of publications he or she produces, as well as where they appear. Journals have become an important part of the academic infrastructure. They play an important role in career routes, both in terms of funding and appointments. Based on a survey conducted among researchers, the primary motivations for publishing their research work were found to be 'advancing my career' and 'securing future funding.' These factors were identified as major drivers for researchers when it comes to publishing their work.

Journals' coverage is frequently selective and specialized. As they compete for articles, their identification acts as a proxy for the research that is published and the significance of that study. The impact factor (a measure of a journal's citations) is commonly viewed as a technique for measuring a journal's value, and it is frequently used (and misused) by writers and academicians to determine where to publish as well as how to rank the importance of a publication.

How to create a frame for a scientific paper?

A paper's format is similar to that of an hourglass (Fig. 1.1), opening wide and then narrowing down to the study's precise topic, hypothesis, methodology, and findings. The discussion and conclusion sections of effective papers broaden the scope of the study by connecting it to the existing literature and showing how the current study would fill a knowledge gap.

Authors publish for several reasons, and the type of article they publish might be quite diverse. Although research articles are commonly associated with journals, there is a wide range of articles that fulfil the objective of communication and provide useful information to the community. News, editorials, letters, reviews, commentaries, photographs, audio clips, and other types of 'articles' can all be beneficial to researchers and can be found in journals.

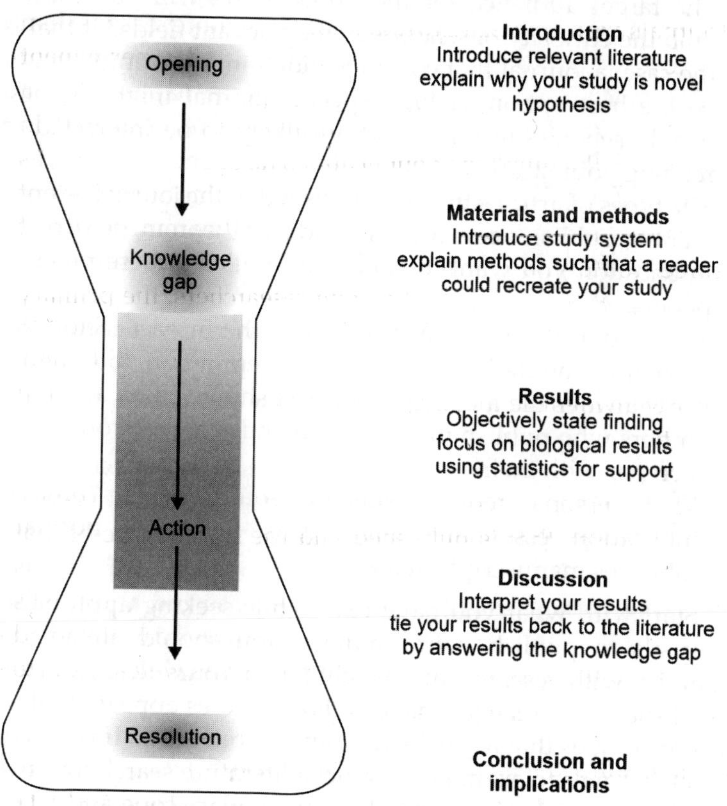

Fig. 1.1: Essential titles for a scientific paper

How to choose a journal?

Submitting a manuscript to the wrong journal is a typical blunder that might result in the paper being rejected even before peer review. Choosing a suitable journal increases the chances of your work being accepted. The following are some things to think about:

- The themes covered by the journal—if your research is in the field of applied science, then submit it to an applied science publication; if it is clinical, then submit it to a clinical journal; and if it is basic research, then submit it to a basic research magazine. You might find it easier to look through a list of journals organized by subject.
- The target audience for the publication—will your study grab the curiosity of scholars in the relevant fields? If that is the case, a journal that covers a wide range of topics would be the best option. A topic-specific journal might be best if only scholars in your field are likely to be interested in reading your study.
- The types of articles that are published in the journal—if you want to publish a review, case study, or theorem, be sure the publication you want to submit it to allows these types of papers.
- The journal's reputation is at stake—the impact factor of a journal is one indicator marking its reputation, although it is not always the most essential. You should think about the authors who publish in the journal and whether your study is on par with theirs.
- What personal requirements do you have—is "time to publication" essential to you, because the journal normally publishes manuscripts quickly?

Start with what you have read while seeking appropriate journals to publish your findings. You should already be familiar with research that is similar to yours that has been published. In which journal did those studies appear? Make a list of journals that might be relevant to your work. If you need more journals to examine, conduct a literature search for other published articles in your field with similar scope and effect, and see where they have been published.

When you have made a list of potential target journals, go to their websites and read what they are saying. Every journal would include a page dedicated to author instructions. Journals on your list that are not a good fit for your work based on the criteria stated above should be excluded. One or more of the remaining journals will almost certainly stand out as an excellent choice. Consider whether conducting more experiments will improve your chances of being published in your preferred journal. If you need to publish quickly, see which of the remaining journals offers rapid publication; if none do, see which has the highest frequency of publication. Consider potential publications that offer an open-access option if your primary goal is to make your work accessible to as many individuals as possible.

Open access allows everyone to view your article online for free, increasing the likelihood that it will be read and cited. It is always a good idea to select your second- and third-choice journals once you have chosen the journal that you think is the best fit for your studies and your goals. If your first-choice publication rejects your manuscript, you can swiftly submit it to your second-choice journal.

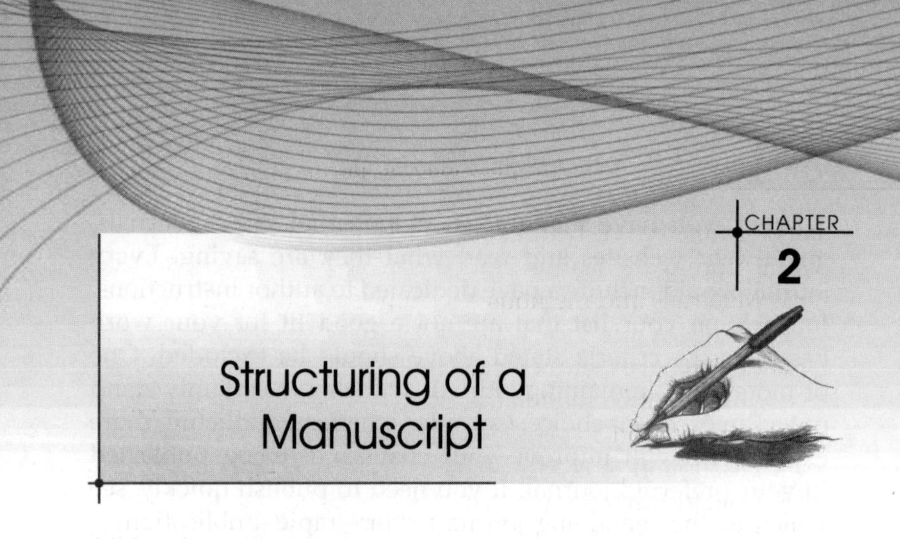

Structuring of a Manuscript

Once you have finished your research, you need to write them up into a cohesive and concise paper that conveys your research's story. Since researchers are time-constrained, research articles must be concise and easy to read. As a result, most papers have a common structure that makes it easy for readers to access the information they need. The usual structure and what to include in each area will be discussed in the following segment.

Outline of IMRaD structure

IMRaD refers to the standard structure of the body of research manuscripts (after the title and abstract), and it refers to,
Introduction
Materials and Methods
Results and
Discussion,
Conclusions

Not all journals use these section titles in this order, but most published articles have a structure similar to IMRaD. This standard structure gives a logical flow to the content, makes journal manuscripts consistent and easy to read, and provides a "map" so that readers can quickly find content of interest in any manuscript. Also, it reminds authors what content should be included in an article. Although the sections of the journal manuscript are published in the order of Title, Abstract, Introduction, Materials and Methods, Results, Discussion, and conclusion, the best and the most recommended approach while drafting the manuscript should be in the following order:

1. Materials and methods
2. Results (write this section first as it is you who has been doing your experiments and collecting the results for it, hence, you would be confident enough to draft these sections).
3. Introduction
4. Discussion
5. Conclusion (after you have had an opportunity to analyze your results and get a feel of their significance, decide on the journal that best suits your study and write these sections next).
6. Title of the article
7. Abstract
8. Keywords (should include the most relevant words which reflects your research topic)

Always, write your title and abstract at the end, after drafting the entire manuscripts, as these are based on all the other sections of your research.

Following this order will help you to write a logical and consistent manuscript.

Also, explain the different sections of your manuscript in a narrative format, similar to that of 'telling a story' on your research and its implications.

The criteria listed below assist potential authors in comprehending the demands of the journal reviewer.

The reviewer's checklist is as follows:

Introduction

- Are the aims/objectives clear?
- Is the importance of the study adequately emphasized?
- Is the subject matter of the study innovative?
- Have the previous works on the relevant subject cited adequately?

Patients (materials) and methods

- Is the study population explained adequately?
- Are the methods clearly described to reproduce the experiment?

- Is the study design clear?
- Have the correct statistical methods/techniques been explained?
- Have the ethical considerations been considered and addressed?

Results

- Can the reader assess the results based on the data obtained?
- Is the data/information straightforward and not confusing?
- Are there adequate controls? (In cases where the study is a case-control/cohort/or RCT study design)
- Have the appropriate statistical methods been used?

Discussion

- Do the authors comment effectively on all their results?
- Have the authors explained why and how their study differs from the previously published ones and have they been cited properly?
- Do the authors discuss the potential problems faced while the study and the limitations of their study?
- Are the author's conclusions supported by the results and consistent with their study's objective?

Suggestions

Tools for writing

- Typeset
- Microsoft word

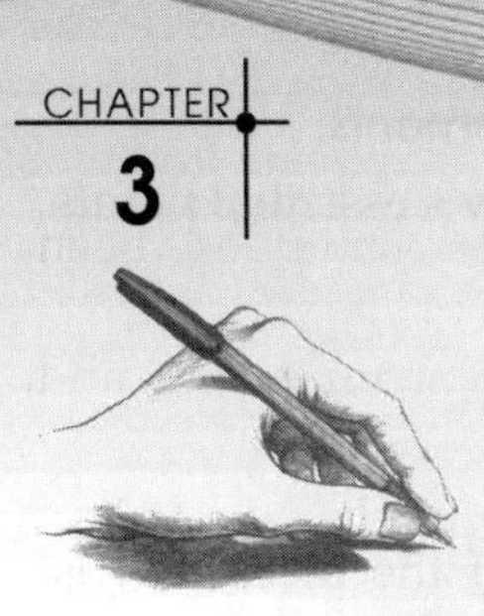

Title, Abstract and Keywords

The "title" and "abstract" of a research paper are the ones which create an initial impression for readers of your research work, so they require careful attention. These are typically composed after completing the entire manuscript, they are of paramount importance because many readers only skim these sections. Hence, the title and abstract should be captivating and succinctly convey the essence of your research.

For the "title," it should be descriptive, direct, correct, relevant, fascinating, concise, exact, unique, and non-misleading. Readers (and reviewers) are frequently introduced to your work through the title of your manuscript. As a result, you must choose a title that catches people's attention, accurately explains the contents of your manuscript, and entices them to read on.

In the case of the "abstract," it should be simple, specific, clear, unbiased, honest, precise, stand-alone, comprehensive, academic, well-structured, and non-misrepresentative. It should align with the main text, particularly after revisions, and should highlight the core message of your research.

Furthermore, it is essential to include crucial keywords within the title and abstract for effective indexing and retrieval in search engines and scientific databases. These keywords should be listed immediately after the abstract to aid in the discoverability of your research. Crafting a compelling title and a well-structured abstract is pivotal to piquing readers' interest and ensuring your research is accessible and appealing to a broader audience.

A good title should include the following elements:

Simple and clear enough to convey the study's essential points
Emphasize the significance of the research
Be succinct.
Attract readers

Significance of the title

The title is the "initial detail" or "face" of the piece that is read when a reader browses through the table of contents of a journal issue (hard copy or online). As a result, it must be straightforward, direct, accurate, appropriate, specific, functional, engaging, appealing, concise/brief, precise/focused, unambiguous, memorable, gripping, informational (enough to entice the reader to continue reading), unique, catchy, and not misleading. It should provide "just enough details" to gain the reader's attention and curiosity, prompting them to read the abstract and, if they are still intrigued, the whole work.

Characteristics of effective titles in academic research papers:

- Indicate accurately the subject and scope of the study.
- Avoiding the use of abbreviations.
- Avoiding the use of any words which would create conflicts.
- Using words that create a positive impression and stimulate the reader's interest.
- Use the current nomenclatures from the field of study.
- Identify key variables, both dependent and independent.
- Reveal how the paper will be organized.
- Suggest a relationship between variables which supports the major hypothesis.
- Is limited to 10–15 substantive words.
- Do include "study of," "analysis of" or similar constructions.
- Titles are usually in the form of a phrase, but can also be in the form of a question.
- Use correct grammar and capitalization, with all first words and last words capitalized, including the first word of a subtitle. All nouns, pronouns, verbs, adjectives, and adverbs that appear between the first and last words of the title are also capitalized.

- In academic papers, rarely is a title followed by an exclamation mark. However, a title or subtitle can be in the form of a question.
- Writing a good title for your manuscript can be challenging. First, list the topics covered by the manuscript. Try to put all of the topics together in the title using as few words as possible.
- A title that is too long will seem clumsy, and monotonous, appear unfocused, annoy readers, and probably not meet journal requirements. While very short titles may not be representational of the contents of the article; hence, the title should be of the ideal length to guarantee that it describes the manuscript's major theme and content.

For example:

Does Vaccinating Adolescents with Influenza Vaccine Inhibit the Spread of Influenza in Unimmunized Residents of Urban Communities?

The above title has too many unnecessary words and does not give enough information about what makes the manuscript interesting.

Effect of Influenza Vaccination on Infection Rates in Urban Communities: A Randomized Trial

Rather, the above is an effective title, as it is short, easy to understand, and conveys the important aspects of the research.

Furthermore, too much technical language or chemical formulas in the title may confuse readers, causing them to skim over the page.

Think about why your research will be of interest to other scientists. This should be related to the reason why you decided to study this topic. If your title makes this clear, it will likely attract more readers to your manuscript.

TIP: Write down a few possible titles, and then select the best to refine further. Ask your colleagues for their opinion. Spending the time needed to do this will result in a better title, which includes, the patients/subjects, design, interventions, comparisons/control, and outcome are all included, but the main result and conclusion are not revealed.

Usually, the descriptive title states the study's primary finding right in the title; it also decreases the reader's curiosity and may indicate author bias; therefore, it should be avoided. Whereas an interrogative title is the one with a research question or an inquiry in the title. A query in the title has the potential to sensationalize the topic and has more downloads (but fewer citations), hence it can be distracting to the reader and is best avoided for a research piece. Therefore, before deciding on a title, it is a good idea to get feedback from peers who are not biased.

Many journals require writers to write a "short title," "running head," or "running title" for use in the printed paper's header or footer. This is a condensed version of the main title that contains up to 40–50 characters and may include standard abbreviations to aid the reader's navigation through the article.

To summarize
The title,
- should be interesting and informative
- should be accurate, specific, and functional
- should be straightforward
- should be concise, and precise, and should include the main theme of the paper
- should not be ambiguous or misrepresentative
- should not be too short or too long
- should avoid strange abbreviations and unnecessary acronyms
- the title should be in PICO style (Population, Intervention, Comparison and Outcome)
- important terms/keywords should be placed at the beginning of the title
- place of the study and sample size should be mentioned only if it adds to the technical value of the title
- descriptive titles are preferred to declarative or interrogative titles
- authors should stick to the word count and other instructions as specified by the target journal

Abstract and Keywords

The abstract is a summary or synopsis of the entire research paper, and it must share many of the same features as the title. It should be straightforward, explicit, functional, clear, unbiased, honest, succinct, exact, self-contained, comprehensive, scholarly, balanced, and not misleading. The abstract is one of the most significant elements of a scientific paper. Successful authors devote a lot of time and attention to their abstracts, which serve as ads for their works. Unfortunately, some authors are unaware of the importance of a strong abstract to the success of their scientific paper.

What is the significance of the abstract?

Most frequently this is the only piece of a document that is read, and it often determines whether a reader will download and read the remaining article. Or, in the case of a conference paper, the abstract will determine whether it is accepted or not for presentation to colleagues. The abstract is an excellent predictor of the quality of the paper, according to conference organizers, journal editors, and reviewers. A sloppy abstract suggests that the author is inexperienced or unconcerned about quality.

It is not difficult to write a good abstract if you know what material to include and how to structure it. You might be unsure about what goes into an abstract if you have never written one before. An abstract should essentially reflect all of the elements in your paper but in a condensed form. In other words, someone reading merely your abstract should be able to grasp why you did the study, how you did it, what you discovered, and why your work is essential. When writing your abstract, avoid the novice's cut-and-paste method and instead develop a distinct, isolated description. Although it is permissible to include data, only report the numbers that indicate the most significant information. Although some authors include citations or URLs in their abstracts, many publications discourage or outright forbid them. Keep in mind that most journals and conferences have a word restriction for abstracts.

Also, think about how to organize your abstract. Some publications or conferences provide a template with four or five sections, such as the background or goal, the question, the methods, the results, and the conclusions. If that is the case, then follow the instructions. If not, the four-part structure outlined below will serve as a good starting point. Your abstract will be well-organized and contain all of the necessary elements if you follow this formula.

The following questions are divided into four sections, each of which requires an answer:

1. **The problem you studied and why is it important?** You should describe the study's background, motivation, and/or the precise topic or hypothesis you addressed in this section. You might be able to set the scene in just one or two sentences, but sometimes a longer description is required. You will have to make your own decisions about how much to convey in this initial section.

2. **What methods did you use to study the problem?** This step is to provide an overview of your methods. Was it a field experiment or a lab experiment? What kinds of treatments were used in the experiments? Unless the techniques section is the emphasis of the work, you should keep it short.

3. **What were the key findings of your research?** Focus on the key finding(s) and provide no more than two or three points when describing your findings. Also, avoid using confusing or imprecise language, which is a common mistake in conference abstracts produced before all the data has been collected and analysed. It should be clear in your mind that," You are not ready to present your paper if your data is incomplete or still being analysed".

4. **What did you summarize based on these findings and what are the broader implications?** The conclusions section is where you should emphasize the study's broader implications. Are the findings novel and innovative? What impact will your results have on the field of study? Do you have any applications? However, do not make broad generalizations that are not backed by evidence or claim that "insights will be explored" in this part.

Therefore, the abstract should highlight the manuscript's selling point and persuade the reader to read the entire work. Keywords (key terms/important words) from all sections of the main content should be used to create the title and abstract. Abstracts are also used when submitting research papers to be considered for presentation at a conference (as oral paper or poster). Grammatical and typographical errors reflect adversely on the quality of the abstract and will show the author's carelessness or casual attitude and should thus be avoided at all costs.

Search Engine Optimization (SEO), which entails including search terms that people are likely to use while looking for articles on your topic, is another crucial consideration when writing an abstract. You should repeat such terms throughout the abstract, in addition to providing them in the title and keyword area of your work. Search engines utilize this type of repetition to rank an online document. You may improve the ranking of your work in a search and make it easier for peers to locate by optimizing your abstract for search engine discovery.

Finally, several journals are now promoting or demanding the use of "enhanced abstracts," such as graphical or video abstracts. Although such abstracts may include extra visual elements, the core requirements remain the same. All good abstracts summarize the paper and include the four critical elements outlined above.

Writing good abstracts is an acquired skill, not an art. It takes time and effort to master such a skill.

Here is a practice activity to help you hone this talent:

- Choose a scientific article relevant to your field.
- Read the paper without looking at the abstract.
- Then, depending on your reading, try to write an abstract.
- Compare and contrast your abstract with the authors.
- Repeat till you are comfortable.

This practice will help you polish the abilities needed to create a short and informative abstract if you have not yet published a paper.

Types of abstract

The abstracts can be structured or unstructured. Most publications prefer structured abstracts since they are more informative and feature specified subheadings/subsections under which the abstract must be written. Context/background, aims, design, setting, participants, interventions, key outcome measures, outcomes, and conclusions are typical subheadings. Some journals follow the IMRaD format for abstract structure, with subheadings such as Introduction/Background, Methods, Results, and (instead of Discussion) Conclusion.

Structured abstracts are preferable because they are more complex, instructive, easier to read, recall, and peer-review; yet, they take up more space and can have the same constraints as an unstructured abstract. Reviewers and readers understand structured abstracts better. In any case, the type of abstract and the subheadings of a structured abstract are determined by the journal style and are not up to the author's discretion. Meta-analysis, educational research, quality improvement activities, reviews, and case studies may require separate subheadings. The CONSORT checklist must be included in clinical trial abstracts. Other types of studies, such as observational studies and investigations of diagnostic accuracy, have similar standards.

Unstructured abstracts are free-flowing, lack pre-defined subheadings, and are frequently used for papers that do not (typically) explain novel research.

The structure of a four-point abstract : The following aspects must be properly balanced about the content/matter beneath each subheading:

Point 1: Background and/or Objectives—this section explains why the work was done and is usually only a few phrases long. This subheading also includes the hypothesis/study question as well as the key objectives.

Point 2: Methods—this section is the most detailed, describing the study design, setting, participants, blinding, sample size, sampling method, intervention(s), length and follow-up, research instruments, key outcome measures, parameters evaluated, and how the outcomes were assessed or analysed.

Point 3: Results—this subsection states what was discovered. This section is longer, harder to write, and must include key facts such as the number of study participants, and analytical results (of primary and secondary objectives), and include the real data.

Point 4: Conclusions—the take-home message (the "so what" of the paper) and other significant/important findings should be mentioned here, considering the interpretation of the research question/hypothesis and results, as well as the author's perspectives on the study's ramifications.

The eight-point structured abstract looks as follows:

Objectives, Study Design, Study Setting, Participants/Patients, Methods/Intervention, Outcome Measures, Results, and Conclusions are the eight subheadings. The journals provide directions to the authors on whether they should use a four- or eight-point abstract, or variations thereof.

Descriptive abstracts: This kind of abstract should be short (75–150 words) and merely describe the contents of the study without offering any additional information; the reader must read the entire manuscript to learn about it. Descriptive abstracts are rarely used for original research papers. These are used for case studies, reviews, and opinions, among other things. Informative abstracts (which can be structured or unstructured, as explained above) provide a detailed explanation of the contents of the paper and accurately reflect the actual research conducted.

Your abstract should answer these questions about your manuscript:

What was done?

Why did you do it?

What did you find?

Why are these findings useful and important?

Answering these questions lets readers know the most important points about your study, and helps them decide whether they want to read the rest of the paper. Make sure you follow the proper journal manuscript formatting guidelines when preparing your abstract.

TIP: Journals often set a maximum word count for abstracts, often 250 words, and no citations. This is to ensure that the full abstract appears in indexing services.

Keywords: These are tools that indexers and search engines use to find publications that are related to them. Readers will be able to find your journal manuscript if database search engines can find it. This will increase the amount of people who read your manuscript, which will almost certainly result in more citations. Keywords, on the other hand, must be properly picked to be effective.

Tips to write a good abstract:
- It should be informative, and cohesive, and adhere to the structure with subheadings provided by the target journal.
- Structured abstracts are preferred over unstructured abstracts
- Should have simple language and phrases
- It should be independent and stand-alone
- It should be concise, interesting, unbiased, precise, honest, and balanced
- It should not be misrepresentative; rather it should be consistent with the main text of the paper
- It should utilize the full-word ability allowed by the journal so that most of the actual scientific facts of the main paper are represented in the abstract
- It should include the key message significantly
- It should adhere to the style and the word count (usually about 250 words) specified by the target journal
- It should avoid abbreviations
- List the appropriate "keywords" below the abstract

To summarize

The abstract is a summary of the content of the journal manuscript
- A time-saving shortcut for busy researchers
- A guide to the most important parts of your manuscript's written content

- Many readers will only read the abstract of your manuscript. Therefore, it must be able to stand alone. In most cases, the abstract is the only part of your article that appears in indexing databases such as Web of Science or PubMed and so will be the most accessed part of your article; making a good impression will encourage researchers to read your full paper.
- A well-written abstract can also help speed up the peer-review process. During peer review, referees are usually only sent the abstract when invited to review the paper. Therefore, the abstract needs to contain enough information about the paper to allow referees to make a judgement as to whether they have enough expertise to review the paper and be engaging enough for them to want to review it.

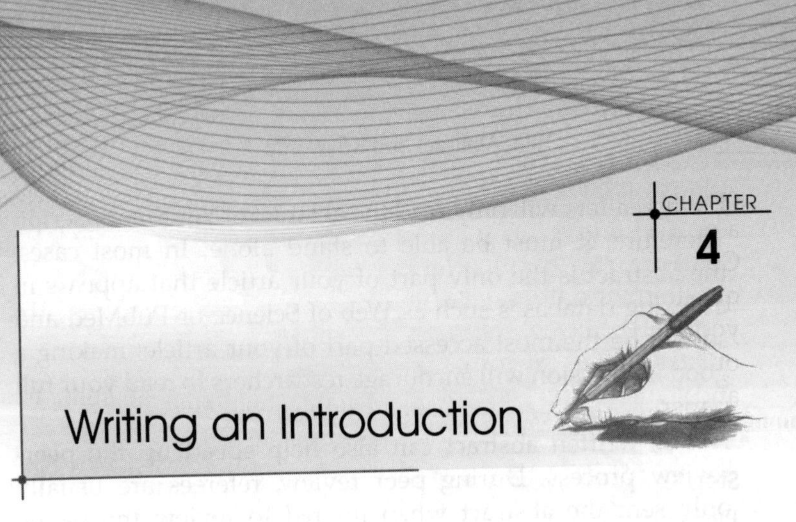

Writing an Introduction

The introduction is to guide the reader from a broad subject area to a specific study field. It establishes the context of the research by summarizing current knowledge and background information on the topic, stating the purpose of the work in the form of a hypothesis, question, or research problem, briefly explaining your rationale, and methodological approach, highlighting the potential outcomes that your study can reveal, and describing the remaining paper's structure. This is the opening to your research paper and this is where you introduce the reader to your topic and strategy.

The main guidelines are as follows:
- Introduce your topic and pique the reader's curiosity.
- Provide background information or a summary of previous studies.
- Create your strategy.
- Describe your research problem in detail.
- Give an overview structure of the paper.

Depending on whether your work discusses the results of unique empirical research or makes a case using several sources, the introduction will be slightly different.

The five steps detailed below will assist you in writing a strong introduction for any form of research paper.

Step 1: How the topic was chosen?

The introduction's initial task is to inform the reader about your topic and why it is fascinating or significant. A strong opening hook is usually used to accomplish this. The hook is a powerful first line that shows the importance of your issue. Consider an intriguing fact or statistic, a powerful remark, a question, or a brief anecdote to pique the reader's interest in your subject. Do not feel like your hook has to be particularly outstanding or inventive. Catchiness is less crucial than clarity and significance. The most important thing is to lead the reader to your topic and place your views in context.

Step 2: Explain your background

Depending on the direction your paper is heading, this section of the introduction will be different. You will go over some general background in a more contentious paper. This is the section of a more empirical study where you review the existing research and determine how yours fits in. Therefore, include only the most important background information. The introduction is not the place to go into great detail; if more background information is required for your paper, it can be included in the body. Instead of detailing original research, you will give a summary of the most relevant research that has previously been done in a paper about original research. This is a condensed version of a literature review, a snapshot of the current state of research on your issue in a few phrases. Genuine interaction with the literature should inform this. While your search may not be as thorough as a full literature review, having a good understanding of the relevant research is critical for informing your work.

Step 3: State your research problem

This stage is to determine where your study fits into the larger picture and what problem it answers. Here, you can simply state the problem you intend to discuss, and what is important about your argument. Relate it to the literature in terms of these questions:

- What is the research gap that your work has planned to fill?
- What are the restrictions of the previous work that it addresses?
- What knowledge contribution does it make?

Step 4: Write your objectives

Set a goal for your research. Now you will go into the details of what you want to learn or say in your research paper. This can be framed in a variety of ways. A thesis statement is presented in an argumentative paper, but a research question is often posed in an empirical paper.

In an empirical research article, the research question is the question you intend to answer. Present your research question simply and directly, with as little elaboration as possible. The rest of the work will be devoted to debating and researching this subject; all you must do now is articulate it. A research question might be explicitly or indirectly framed. If you tested hypotheses as part of your research, make sure to mention them alongside your research question. Because the hypothesis will have already been tested by the time you write your article, and they are frequently provided in the past tense.

A quick synopsis of the rest of the article is frequently included in the introduction's closing section. This is not essentially required in a publication that follows the usual scientific format of "introduction, methodology, results, and discussion." It is crucial to define the shape of your article to the reader if it is structured less predictably.

While writing the background, make sure your citations are:

- Well-balanced: If experiments have found conflicting results on a question, ensure that you have cited studies with both kinds of results.
- Current literature: Every research discipline is different, but you should aim to cite references that are not more than 10 years old if possible. However, be sure to cite the first discovery or mention in the literature even if it is older than 10 years.
- Relevant: This is the most important requirement. The studies you cite should be strongly related to your research question.

TIP: Do not write a literature review in your introduction, but do cite reviews where readers can find more information if they want it.

Once you have provided background material and stated the problem or question for your study, tell the reader the purpose of your study. Usually, the reason is to fill a gap in the knowledge or to answer a previously unanswered question. For example, if a drug is known to work well in one population, but has never been tested in a different population, the purpose of a study could be to test the efficacy and safety of the drug in the second population.

The final thing to include at the end of your introduction is a clear and exact statement of your study aims. You might also explain in a sentence or two about how you conducted the study.

To summarize: Important factors to keep in mind include
- Following the explanations in the 'Introduction' section, abbreviations should be used (their explanations in the summary do not count)
- Present tense should be employed in it is the simplest form.
- Updated publications having a higher impact factor, as well as prestigious source books, should be used as references.
- Avoid enigmatic and perplexing terms; instead, use plain statements that address troublesome issues and their answers.
- The sentences should be appealing, intriguing, and easy to understand.

Writing Methods

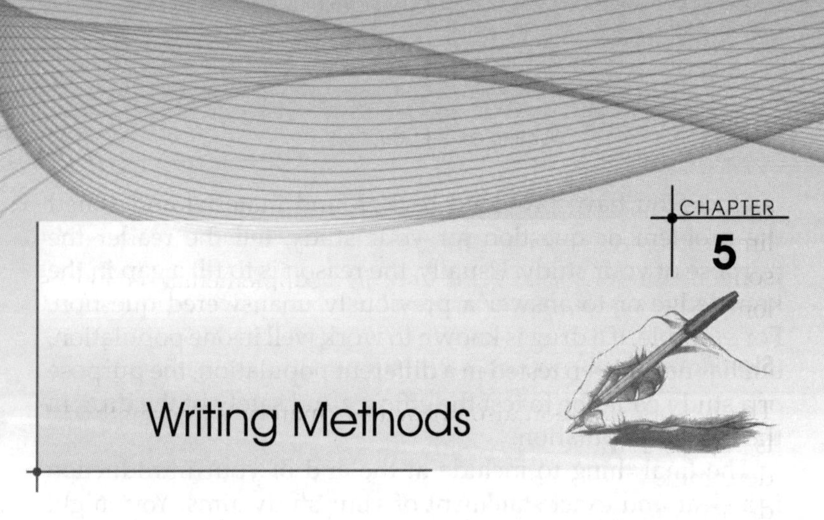

An explanation of the processes used to experimenting the study is included in the Methods section of the research article. The goal for authors of scientific research articles is to convey their findings clearly and succinctly while still providing enough information to allow the experiment to be replicated. The methods section is the most important aspect of a research paper because it provides the information by which the validity of a study is ultimately judged. Therefore, the author must provide a clear and precise description of how an experiment was done and the rationale for the specific experimental procedures chosen. A clear methodology section serves as the foundation for promoting openness and replicability in research. Its clarity not only influences how editors evaluate the work but also enhances reader comprehension.

The Materials and Methods section should contain enough information for the researchers to understand your work in such a way that it will allow appropriately trained investigators to fully replicate your research. However, there is no need to go into the level of detail that a layperson would require, as the reader is also trained in your profession and has the necessary skills and knowledge to attempt a replication. A consistent principle of rigorous, transparent, and Open Science is to provide a methods section that allows other researchers to understand and duplicate your findings. While not every diary entry is essential for inclusion in this section, it is crucial to prioritize thoroughness, as ensuring reproducibility remains an essential responsibility for the author. By exceeding a minimum standard of knowledge, you cannot cause any complications. It is fine if a publication still has a word limit, either for the entire article or for a certain section and needs some methodological details to be in a supplemental section, as long as the extra information is searchable.

Significance of method section

The Methods section also known as "materials and methods" is crucial because it gives the reader enough information to determine whether the study is valid and repeatable. Figure 5.1 depicts the guidelines for writing this section and this can be used to verify if you are drafting the method section correctly.

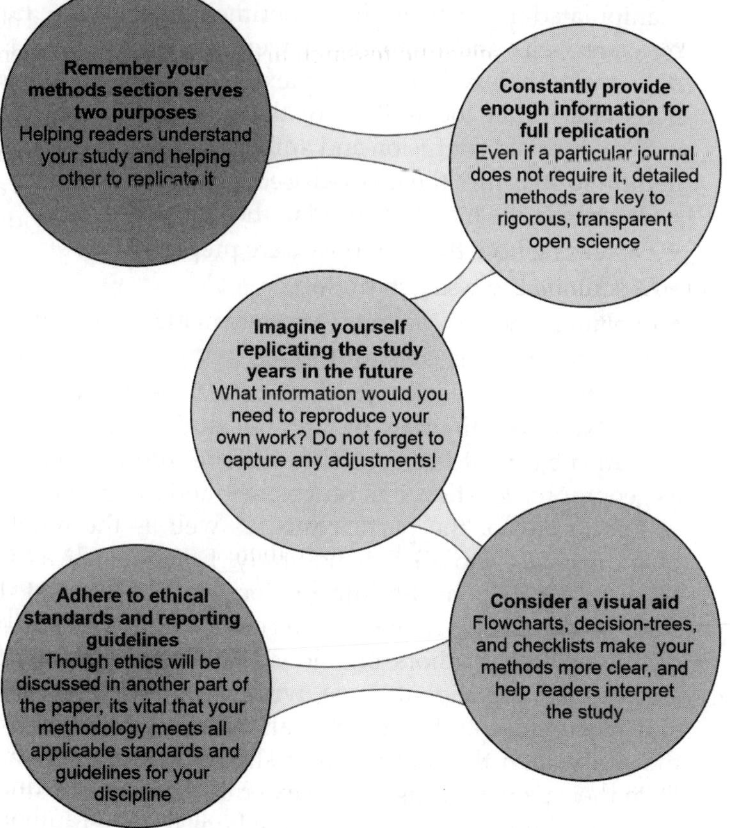

Fig. 5.1: Guidelines in writing methods

Writing Style of the Methods Section

The following is a list of important sections that should be included in a research paper's methods section; writers may utilize subheadings to describe their research more clearly.

1. **Search the literature:** Authors should cite all the sources that aided in their method selection. It is mandatory to include the dates of previous experiments as well as their specific specifications. "Materials" refer to what was examined (e.g. humans, animals, samples used, tissue preparations) and the various treatments (e.g. drugs, gases) and instruments (e.g., X-ray, CT scan, ventilators) used in the study. "Methods" refer to, how subjects or objects were manipulated to answer the experimental question, how measurements and calculations were made, and how the data were analyzed. The complexity of scientific inquiry necessitates that the writing of the methods is clear and orderly to avoid confusion and ambiguity. First, it is usually helpful to structure the methods section by:
   - Describing the materials used in the study
   - Explaining how the materials were prepared
   - Describing the research protocol
   - Explaining how measurements were made
   - What calculations were performed
   - Statistical tests which were done to analyze the data

2. **Study samples (human or animal study):** When using human subjects: It is essential to include information such as geographic location, age ranges, sex, and medical history (if applicable) of the participants, as well as the number of individuals chosen for the study. Details such as the individual's basic health information and vital data at the start of the study, if hospital records were used should be mentioned. Authors should additionally declare that each study participant gave written informed consent, and when children below 18 years of age are involved in the study, then the consent form should be duly obtained from their parents. Judging the external validity of a study involving human subjects (i.e. to whom the study results may be applied) requires that descriptive data be provided

regarding the basic demographic profile of the sample population, including age, gender, and possibly the racial composition of the sample. When reviewing and evaluating patient records, authors should state whether the reviewers were blinded to them.

When using animal subjects: Authors should cite the source of any non-human subjects that were used in their study. The number of animals utilized, their species, weight, strain, ages, genders, and initial conditions, as well as how they were kept and cared for, should all be documented. Details of any special equipment utilized, such as housing and feeding requirements should be included.

In general, authors should explain their inclusion and exclusion criteria of study subjects, including how they were decided and how many subjects were excluded. It is also mandatory to explain how the chosen group was separated into subgroups and their features, as well as the control group.

The method section should utilize subheadings to divide up different subsections. These subsections typically include participants, materials, design, and procedure.

a. **Participants:** In this part of the method section, you should describe the participants in your experiment including who they were, how many were there, how they were selected and any unique features that may set them apart from the general population. Also, should explain how many participants were assigned to each condition, and the basic characteristics of your participants such as sex, age, ethnicity, or religion. In this subsection, it is also important to explain why your participants took part in your research. Was your study advertised at a college or hospital? Did participants receive some types of incentive to take part in your research? Be sure to explain how participants were assigned to each group. Were they assigned randomly to a condition or was some other selection method used? Information on participants helps other researchers understand how your study was performed, how generalizable the result might be, and allows other researchers to replicate your results with other populations to see if they might obtain the same results.

b. **Materials:** Describe the materials, measures, equipment, or stimuli used in the experiment. This may include testing instruments, technical equipment, books, images, or other materials used during research. If you have used some type of psychological assessment or special equipment were used while carrying out your experiment, it should be noted in this part of your method section.

c. **Design:** Describe the type of design used in the experiment. Specify the variables as well as the levels of these variables. Identify your independent variables, dependent variables, control variables, and any extraneous variables that might influence your results. Explain whether your experiment uses a within-groups or between-groups design.

d. **Procedure:** This section should detail the procedures used in your experiment. Explain what you had participants do, how you collected data and the order in which the steps occurred. Authors should discuss how they conducted their research. Instruments and any necessary preparations (e.g. blood or tissue samples, medications) must be discussed.

3. **Statistical analyses:** The appropriate use of statistical tools and analysis, in addition to clear procedures and transparent study design, has an impact on editorial judgement and readers' knowledge and faith in science. The type of data, how it was measured, and the statistical tests used should all be reported along with the version of the statistical tool used. Must remember that this is not the "results" section; any pertinent tables and figures should be cited afterwards. Mention which software was used for analysis along with its version. The statistical methods must never be manipulated or misapplied. A serious ethical infraction involves misrepresenting data, selectively reporting results, or hunting for patterns that can be portrayed as statistically significant to arrive

at a conclusion that is thought to be more deserving of attention or publishing. Using statistics to "spin" data, while seemingly innocent, might prevent publication, weaken a published work, or lead to an investigation and retraction.

4. **Ethical consideration:** It is just as crucial to assure readers that you followed all relevant ethical norms when performing your research as it is to describe what you did. While ethical standards and reporting rules are frequently included in a distinct section of a study, make sure your procedures and protocols adhere to these standards.

For Systematic Reviews and Meta-Analyses

Preferred Reporting Items for Systematic Reviews and Meta-Analyses (PRISMA) is an evidence-based minimal set of items for reporting reviews of randomized trials and other types of research.

For Randomized Controlled Trials (RCT)

The Consolidated Standards of Reporting Trials (CONSORT) project encompasses several projects aimed at preventing difficulties with randomized controlled trials reporting. The main endeavour is the CONSORT statement, which is an evidence-based minimal set of recommendations for reporting randomized trials.

The Animal Research

Reporting of *in vivo* experiments standards encourages researchers to record as much information as possible in animal research, reducing the number of superfluous studies.

To summarize

Do's

- Keep future replicability in mind, as well as comprehension and readability.
- Follow checklists and criteria specific to the field and journal.
- Consider making a personal commitment to rigorous and transparent science, rather than simply following journal norms.

- Determine whether any research resources you utilize have persistent identifiers that can be specifically cited in your methods section.
- Make a list of all decisions taken during the experiments that someone who wants to replicate your work would need to know about.
- Create a permanent link to your laboratory procedures by storing them on the protocols.io website. You, as well as future scientists who follow your methods, can update them if you enhance them.

Don'ts
- Summarize or abbreviate methods without providing comprehensive details in a supplemental section that can be found.
- Assume you will always remember how you did things, or that you will have access to private or institutional notebooks and resources.
- Attempt to conceal any limit or suboptimal decisions you have to make transparency is the key to assuring your research's legitimacy.

Finally, if you are writing your paper for a class or a specific publication, be sure to keep in mind any specific instructions provided by your instructor or by the journal editor. Your instructor may have certain requirements that you need to follow while writing your method section. Authors should avoid providing extensive details or an exhaustive list of equipment used, as readers may become distracted. This extraneous information does little to support the research and does not assist the reader in understanding how the goal was met. One of the most significant sections of the paper is the methods section. Authors should keep in mind that they should always prepare a draft that lists all elements, let others examine it, and rewrite it to remove any unnecessary material.

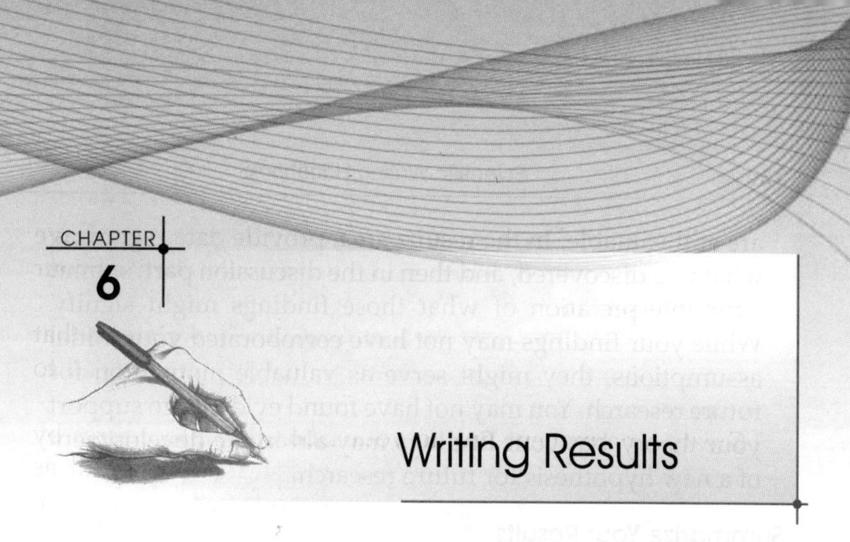

Writing Results

The results section summarizes the data that was collected and the statistical analyses that were performed. The goal of this section is to report the results without any type of subjective interpretation.

Here is how you have to write a results section of your paper:

- The results should justify your claims—to adequately substantiate your conclusions, you must report data. Because you will be discussing your interpretation of the results in the discussion section, you should be sure that the data in the results section supports your claims. Look back over your findings section as you compose your discussion section to make sure you have all the information you need to adequately support your conclusions.

- Do not omit relevant findings—your results section should not only adequately substantiate your claims, but it should also present a realistic picture of what you discovered in your research. Make sure to include all pertinent information. If your hypothesis called for more statistically significant outcomes, do not throw out the results if they do not match your expectations.

- Negative outcomes should not be overlooked—it does not mean a result is not significant just because it does not support your theory. Results that contradict your theory can be just as instructive as those that do. Even if your research did not confirm your hypothesis, the results you reached are still valuable. In the results area, provide data regarding what you discovered, and then in the discussion part, submit your interpretation of what those findings might signify. While your findings may not have corroborated your initial assumptions, they might serve as valuable motivation for future research. You may not have found evidence to support your theory, but your findings may aid in the development of a new hypothesis for future research.

Summarize Your Results

The raw data should not be included in the results section. Remember that you are summarizing the findings rather than reporting them in depth. The results section should be a concise summary of your findings rather than a detailed breakdown of every single figure and calculation. You can build an additional online archive if you choose, where other scholars can access the raw data if they want to.

Illustrations (tables and figures)

- Both text and illustrations should be included in your results section—the reader will be able to easily glance at your results if you present the data in this manner.
- Figures and tables (display items) are frequently the most efficient way to convey enormous amounts of complex information that would be difficult to describe through words.
- Display pieces are also crucial for drawing readers' attention to your work as readers will be compelled to take the time to study a figure if it is well-designed and appealing, and they may even be enticed to read the entire work if it is well-designed and attractive.

  Many readers will simply look at your display elements and skip over your manuscript's primary material. As a result, make sure your display items can stand alone from the text and properly explain your most important findings.
- Professionally crafted display elements add a polished touch to your work, instilling an impression of professionalism. A scientifically presented paper gives the impression of

containing robust science, thereby leading readers to perceive it as high-quality. As a result, readers may be more inclined to believe your findings and interpretations.

Consider the following questions when deciding which of your findings to publish as display items:
- Is there any information that you think readers would prefer to see as a display item rather than text?
- Do your figures add to the text rather than duplicate what you have already said?
- Have you included data in a table that can be simply described in the text, such as simple statistics or p values?

Tables

Tables are a great method to convey a lot of information in a short amount of time. You should carefully plan them so that you can effectively communicate your findings to busy researchers.

An example of a well-designed table is as follows:
- The legend/caption should be clear and simple.
- For clarity, data can be separated into groups (if necessary).
- Check if there is enough space between the columns and rows.
- Ensure that the units available are mentioned appropriately.
- The font type and size are both readable and based on journal instructions.

Figures

Just like tables, all figures necessitate to have a clear and succinct legend caption to accompany them.

Figures are ideal for presenting in the following formats:
- Chart/graph
- Images
- Data plots
- Maps
- Schematics

Images

Readers can visualize the information you are trying to impart with the use of images. It is not always easy to be appropriately descriptive with words. Images can aid in the precision required for a scientific publication. It would be good in this scenario to provide a microscope image.

For images, be sure to include:

- Scale bars—label the essential items, indicate the meaning of different colours and symbols used
- Data charts—make it simple to express large volumes of information. The goal is usually to show a functional or statistical relationship between two or more objects. Individual data points, on the other hand, are typically overlooked in favour of concentrating on the relationship revealed by the collection of points.
- Data plots—label all the axes, label all curves and data sets, use a legible font size and specify units for quantities.

Maps

Field work must be placed in the context of the site where it was done, hence maps are essential. A decent map will aid your reader in comprehending how the site impacts your research. It will also assist other researchers in replicating your findings or locating other areas with similar qualities.

For maps, be sure to:

- include latitude and longitude
- include scale bars
- label important items
- consider adding a map legend

Schematics

Schematics assist in identifying the critical components of a system or process. They should only highlight the most significant components, as adding unnecessary items can lead the image to become cluttered. A schematic just contains the drawings that the author chooses, giving it more flexibility than photos. They can also be utilized in situations where taking a picture is difficult or impossible.

For schematics, be sure to:

- Label key items,
- provide complementary explanations in the caption and main text.

TIP 1: It is important to consider how your figures will look in print as well as online. A resolution of 72 ppi is sufficient for online publication whilst in print 100 ppi is recommended. You can adjust the resolution of your figure within the original program you used to create it at the time you saved the file.

TIP 2: There are two main colour models; RGB which stands for red, green, blue and CMYK which stands for cyan, magenta, yellow and black. Most microscopes will take images using the RGB, however, CMYK is the standard used for printing so it is important to check that your figures will display well in this format.

Avoiding image manipulation

You should never intentionally alter your pictures to influence or better your outcomes. You should only minimally process your figures before submitting them to the journal to minimize unintended tampering; your supplied photos should authentically replicate the original image files. In fluorescence microscopy, adjusting the brightness or contrast of an image is only permissible if it is done consistently across all images, including the controls. Cropping photos in the construction of figures should be avoided unless it improves the presentation's clarity and conciseness significantly. Make sure that any vital information for interpreting the figure is not cropped out, such as molecular markers in electrophoresis gels. Any modifications or software that was utilized should be mentioned.

TIP: Keep copies of the original images, files and metadata used to create your figures as these can be requested by the journal during the review process.

Your results section should be organized around tables or figures that summarize the findings of your statistical research. In many circumstances, the simplest method to accomplish this is to build your tables and figures first, and then logically organize them. Then, to accompany your illustrated resources, produce a summary text. If you are not going to talk about tables and figures in the body text of your results section, then do not include them. In your illustrative materials, do not repeat the same data and information presented earlier. Do not provide data in a figure if it has already been presented in a table. If you have already shown data in a figure, do not show it in a table.

Report Your Statistical Findings

Always presume that your audience is well-versed in statistical principles, hence just give the results without explaining what a t-test is or how a one-way ANOVA works. It is not your obligation to teach your readers how to evaluate or interpret statistics; rather, it is your responsibility to report the findings of your research.

Include Effect Sizes

The Publication Manual of the American Psychological Association (APA) recommends including effect sizes in the results section so that readers can appreciate the importance of your study's findings.

To Summarize

Here are a few more tips for writing a results section

- The results section should be written in the past tense.
- Focus on being concise and objective. You will have the opportunity to give your interpretations of the results in the discussion section.
- Read more information on how to write a results section based on the journal style.
- Visit your library and read some journal articles that are on your topic. Pay attention to how the authors present the results of their research.
- Remember, the results section of your paper is all about simply providing the data from your study. This section is often the shortest part of your paper, and in most cases, the most clinical. Be sure not to include any subjective interpretation of the results. Simply relay the data most objectively and straightforwardly as possible. You can then provide your analysis of what these results mean in the discussion section of your paper.

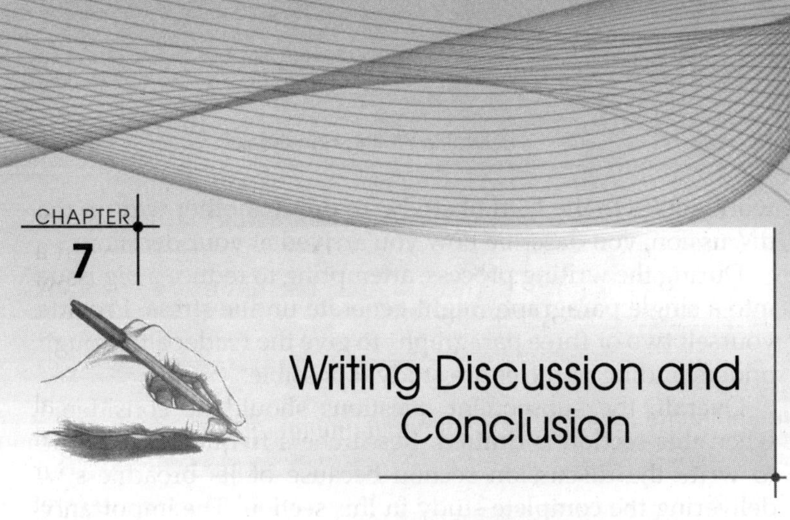

Writing Discussion and Conclusion

The introduction and the debate should complement each other. The introduction starts with a broad focus and concludes with a narrow focus, whereas the discussion starts with a narrow focus (your findings) and ends with a broad focus (the current study) (contextualizing your findings to the field at large). In the discussion part, many of the elements from the introduction section are employed in reverse order and these elements are frequently utilized to interpret results, but in the introduction, they are used to orient the reader within the current state of study. In the discussion section, the findings of the study and conclusions are provided which is a well-written commentary showing the readers what they can learn from your research and contextualize the results.

The discussion section usually necessitates the most consideration because it is here that you interpret your findings. Your discussion should be a separate chapter that connects the introduction and results sections. One method for writing the discussion is to begin by describing the key findings of your research(s). Also, remind the reader of the knowledge gap highlighted in the introduction to revive the interest in the issue you set out to cover. Then, particularly outline how your experiment advanced the discipline by closing a knowledge gap.

The substance of the discussion section is more difficult to define than the other sections. According to the discussion, the study results are described as well as the contributions the work makes to the field of study. To put it another way, in the discussion, you describe how you arrived at your decision.

During the writing process, attempting to reduce a big issue into a single paragraph might generate undue stress. Provide yourself two or three paragraphs to give the reader a thorough understanding of the entire study if possible.

Overall, the subsequent questions should be considered when this section is drafted. Researchers frequently struggle to write the discussion section because of its broadness in delivering the complete study in this section. The importance of the findings is usually overlooked or understated. Even if the data in a study is valid and exciting, a poor interpretation of the data may cause a journal editor or reviewers to reject the submission. Many young researchers make the common mistake of restricting the discussion to a comparison of their findings to those of others.

In addition to these mistakes, you should do the following when writing a discussion (essential content in the discussion section):

- Prepare an outline to organize your thoughts in a logical order as a first step in producing this section.
- Keep the objective/hypothesis of your study in mind while writing to avoid obscuring your message with other concerns.
- Consider utilizing subheadings to highlight the important ideas you want the reader to take as a take-home message from a long conversation.

Figure 7.1 provides a roadmap to write this discussion section.

After the first paragraph of your discussion, we propose responding to your question and hypotheses with specific evidence from your results. Set out each competing explanation in detail if a finding has multiple possible interpretations. To avoid plagiarising, write the discussion in your own words after understanding, summarising, and generalizing relevant literature. Use the first person and active voice to make your debate livelier and more interesting. Even if you are the only one who wrote this section, you should use the word "we." Use

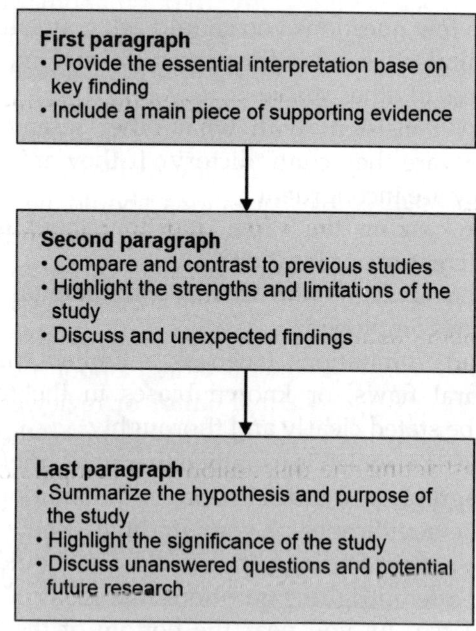

Fig. 7.1: Content for writing discussion

the past tense to allude to your discoveries, and the present tense to refer to broad information. Use the present tense when responding to questions or describing the significance of your study. Use the present perfect to express what you have accomplished during the writing process (for example, "we have described").

Each author presents the discussion section in a different order. So, a format for discussion sections was proposed to increase consistency. This framework, helps the reader locate the specific content in the discussion and tells the writer of the most important topics to address in this section. As per this format, the discussion section will start with concrete facts and ends with broad statements. While this framework is not a "one-size-fit is-all" formula, it may assist new researchers in more efficiently preparing this important component of a scientific study. In addition to this, it is recommended to refer to previous literature and explain how your findings relate to earlier discoveries.

Here are a few questions you should ask yourself:

- What similarities and differences do my findings have with those of other studies?
- Are they consistent with what other researchers have found, or are they contradictory? If they are, talk about why they are incongruent.
- Are you, asking the same question about a different system, creature, or location?
- Was there a distinction in the experimental design or procedures employed?
- Any study limitations (such as a limited sample size, procedural flaws, or known biases in the techniques) should be stated clearly and thoroughly.

The conclusion, which is usually either in its brief section or the last paragraph of the discussion, is the final opportunity to convey the significance of your findings. Rather than just restating your main findings, the conclusion should integrate new ideas or offer intriguing questions that occurred as a result of your research. As you near the bottom of the hourglass, broaden your point of view once again. While it is required to address the study project's faults or cautions, do so near the beginning of the conclusion or earlier in the discussion.

Statement of principal findings

Begin by briefly restating the major findings of your research(s). To answer the study question/purpose, the major finding(s) should use the same key terms as the introduction. If the research question was only partially answered, explain which components of the research question were answered and why. The study's conclusion is the answer to the research question. As a result, it should be mentioned at the beginning of the discussion and used to launch a discussion of the results' broader implications or generalizations. Following the pertinent results, you should provide supporting evidence or other notable findings (positive or negative).

Alternatively, you can start the discussion section before presenting your main findings by reiterating key points from the introduction and/or material and methods sections to help readers understand the context of your research.

The discussion, for example, begins with general information gleaned from the introduction: The authors then describe information gaps, which are typically mentioned in the introduction: "... although no research has been previously addressed ..." or "has not been proven in full yet." Another approach is for the authors to begin the discussion by reminding the reader of the information presented in the material and methods part: For example, the study's goal ("The goal of this study was ...") is described, followed by a discussion of data from the material and methods section. The essential results are presented in these four examples after a contextualization: "... we show that ...", "... we discovered that ...", "... this work demonstrate that ...", and "The results for ...".

Strengths and weaknesses of the study

In this section, you must highlight the benefits and drawbacks (or limitations) of your methodology and approach. While the study's strengths can help readers trust the validity of the conclusions obtained, editors and readers are more interested in the study's flaws. As a result, give both strengths and constraints equal weight. The assumption is that there is no evidence to refute your hypothesis and that the experimental design used is reasonable when discussing limitations.

You can be sure that if you do not criticize your study, the reviewers will. We present study restrictions in papers for ethical and practical reasons. Limitations are useful since they show readers which "mistakes" we made so they do not repeat them. You must explain why the limit is/was discovered, as well as the implications of these constraints for the findings of your investigation. You might even recommend adjustments to the study design to help future studies avoid "mistakes."

Discuss the strengths and disadvantages in comparison to previous studies, with a focus on any discrepancies in findings. After you have given your core findings and addressed the strengths and weaknesses of your study, the next stage is to extend the debate by commenting on your study's key findings concerning other studies in the literature. Limit your discussion to pertinent research in your field of expertise.

Although research not covered in the introduction can be mentioned in the discussion, it is unusual to make a first-time reference to a large number of studies.

Your research could either confirm (for which you could write: Our research confirms ..., our findings are consistent with ...) or refute (which can be written as our research differs from ..., but other studies have revealed that ...) the present state of knowledge. Your study can also add to (our study adds ...) or extend the results of prior studies (our study extends ...). It can also modify knowledge in a specific area (our study modifies ...). You should also explore how the findings of other studies could be merged with your findings to gain a greater understanding of the topic at hand, or you could offer an improved or new model. Also, consider drawing a diagram to help explain the model and, if necessary, outline how to validate it.

Your study's strengths in comparison to those of other studies may help you persuade your readers of the quality of your research and the validity of your conclusion but do not hide what your study's limit is. Knowing your study's limit might help you minimize your results' generalizations and identify methods to improve future studies. You will persuade your readers more if you outline and specify future strategies to employ. Unless you make so many mistakes that your results become inaccurate, then you have undoubtedly gained knowledge from your research.

Compare your material and methods section to those of previous research when outlining the strengths and limitations of your study. In general, disparities in outcomes can be explained by the methods used to obtain them. If you are stumped as to why the results are contradictory, say: We are stumped as to why .... When it is appropriate, you should explain any assumptions (or premises) you have made up front so that the research's validity can be judged. Unexpected results should be discussed as well. If the study was well-run, outcomes that differed from expectations must be interpreted. These findings may lead to discoveries shift the focus of your research, or act as useful indicators for knowledge growth.

When unexpected findings change the emphasis of your research, you should inform the reader (to our surprise ..., surprisingly ...) and briefly summarize your surprising findings neutrally and subjectively.

It is certainly challenging to write a discussion section for the first time. Even for seasoned authors, the first draft of the discussion is likely to undergo numerous revisions as the text "develops." Nevertheless, practising and evaluating are essential for increasing discussion writing skills, just as they are for any other activity in life.

TIP: We would like to leave you with two pieces of advice: firstly, try to review manuscripts written by colleagues to build a capacity to analyze (separate components of manuscripts to better assess each section), and secondly, read as many papers as you can, critically, to learn how important scientific groups communicate results and discuss them.

When writing a discussion, researchers should consider the subject under inquiry, the quality of the work done, and what might be changed in future investigations. It is not easy to master scientific writing, but it may be a pleasant experience for both rookie and seasoned authors.

In brief, a discussion should be organized information in the following order:

a. The study's strengths and limitations;

b. The study's strengths and flaws in comparison to other studies, focusing on any differences in results;

c. The study's meaning: Probable mechanisms and implications; and

d. Scope for outstanding questions and future research.

To summarize

A well-written discussion section places your findings in context, for which the following items should be included:

• The results of your research.

• A review of existing research.

• A comparison of your results to your original hypothesis.

- Discuss your findings in the order of importance from most to least.
- Compare your findings to those of other studies to see if they are consistent. If not, talk about what could be causing the discrepancy.
- Mention any outcomes that are not conclusive and explain them as best you can.
- Also, you could recommend other experiments to help clarify your findings.
- Briefly outline your study's limit to demonstrate to reviewers and readers that you have examined the flaws in your experiment. Many researchers are afraid to do this because they believe it exposes their research's flaws to the editor and reviewer. This, on the other hand, gives your work a favourable impression by demonstrating that you have a thorough comprehension of your issue and can think objectively about your research.
- Discuss the implications of your findings for researchers in your field, researchers in other fields, and the general public.
- Mention how might your discoveries be put to use.
- Describe how your findings add to the findings of past research. If your findings are tentative, make recommendations for future research.
- Finally, at the end of your discussion and conclusions sections, state the most important conclusions of your research once again.

Conclusion Section

The conclusion is usually included (as the final piece) in the discussion section. You must include a brief explanation of your findings as well as their implications for your wide study topic. Most journals do not require a separate conclusion section. For those who do, you should put this under a different heading.

What should you do?

- Read the guidelines for the discussion and conclusion sections as mentioned in the journal. Learn about the guidelines as much as possible before writing the conversation to guarantee you are writing to their specifications.

- Begin with a concise summary of the main findings. This will reaffirm the reader's major takeaway and establish the tone for the rest of the debate.
- Explain why the reader should care about the results of your investigation. Discuss the implications of your findings in light of earlier research, stressing both the research's strengths and shortcomings.
- State if the results support or refute your hypothesis. What could be the causes for your idea being disproved?
- Introduce new or enlarged perspectives on the research problem.
- Indicate what steps should be taken next to address any unanswered questions.
- If you are dealing with a current or ongoing issue, such as climate change, or COVID-19, then talk about the implications of avoiding the situation.
- Be succinct. Adding extraneous information can detract from the core conclusions.

Should not do the following in discussion

- Rewriting your abstract if necessary. In general, statements that begin with "we investigated" or "we studied" do not fit in a conversation.
- Including new arguments or evidence that has not been discussed previously. The primary body of the document should include all necessary information and evidence.
- Do not undercut your credibility by inserting assertions that cast doubt on your technique or execution. Therefore, apologize, even if your study has serious flaws.
- Avoid discussing restrictions or poor outcomes. Readers will gain a thorough comprehension of the provided study if the limit is limited and bad results are included.

Suggested software to check for grammar in writing research work:
- Grammarly
- White smoke

- Scribendi
- Linguix
- Best grammar checker.
- Ref-n-Write
- ProWritingAid
- Quill bot
- Write check
- MS Office's Word Editor grammar tool

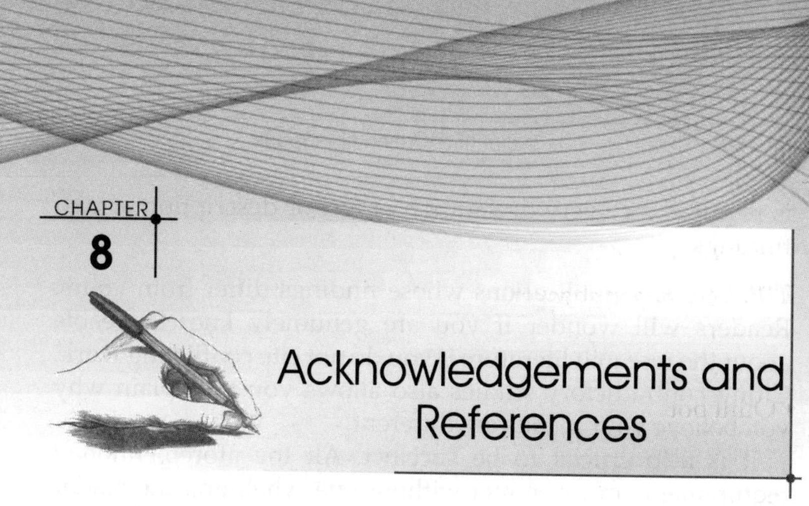

Acknowledgements and References

Acknowledgements

This section normally comes after the sections on discussion and conclusions. The goal is to recognize and acknowledge everyone who participated in the research but did not qualify for authorship. Recognize anybody who helped with ideas, technical assistance (including writing and editing), or special equipment or resources.

TIP: Every Journal Editor offer detailed rules for scientists in all domains on who to list as an author and who to add in the Acknowledgements. Some journals request that you use this section to provide information about funding by including specific grant numbers and titles. Check your target journal's instructions for authors for specific instructions. If you need to include funding information, list the name(s) of the funding organization(s) in full, and identify which authors received funding for what.

References

This is one of the sections which is not paid much attention to. There is also a common misconception that the more references quoted more will be the chances of acceptance of the article, however, this is not true. References should be given equal importance as that of the remaining article.

Failure to adequately acknowledge other works can lower your chances of being published, as references play a crucial role in many aspects of a manuscript. A supporting reference is required for every declaration of fact or description of past findings.

TIP: Cite any publications whose findings differ from yours. Readers will wonder if you are genuinely knowledgeable about the research literature if you do not cite conflicting work. Citing contradictory studies also allows you to explain why you believe your results are different.

It is also crucial to be succinct. All the aforementioned requirements must be met without overwhelming the reader with too many references—only the most relevant and recent publications should be quoted. Although there is no set number of references for an article, check the journal's rules to see if there are any restrictions on the number of references.

TIP: Never mention a publication just based on what you have read in another publication (such as a review) or the abstract alone. These could lead you and your readers astray. Read the article before citing it, and double-check the citation's accuracy before submitting your manuscript.

You must reference other works to:

- **Establish the source of ideas**
  It is crucial to tell your readers who came up with an idea or thought when you mention it. You offer credit to the authors and help others judge the relevance of individual publications by acknowledging publications that have inspired your work. An important ethical concept is to acknowledge the contributions of others.

- **Validate claims**
  All statements in a scientific manuscript must be backed up by evidence. This proof could originate from current study findings, common knowledge, or prior publications. When a claim is accompanied by a citation, it is evident which previous study supports the assertion.

- **Provide a framework for your work**
  Citations assist indicate how a paper fit is into the better picture of scientific study by highlighting similar works. Readers will better appreciate the magnitude of your work

if they know what prior research has discovered and what problems or debates your study is related to.

- **Show there is interest in your field of research**
  Citations show that other researchers are performing work similar to your own. Having current citations will help journal editors see that there is a potential audience for your manuscript. In-text citations, reference list entries, and (occasionally) the layout of your article are all governed by different citation styles. Because the variations can be subtle, it is crucial to double-check the guidelines of the style you are employing.

You must include a reference in the text when you refer to a source (for example, by citing or paraphrasing). Citations can be divided into three categories, namely:

a. **Parenthetical citation:** In your writing, you put the source reference in parentheses. The author's last name, as well as the publishing date and/or page number, are generally included.
b. **Note citation:** In a footnote or endnote, you cite the source.
c. **Numeric citation:** In your reference list, number each of your sources and use the correct number when citing them.

You include a list of all the sources you cited at the end of your work. Each entry in the list corresponds to an in-text citation and provides complete publication information so that the reader may quickly locate the source.

The name of this list varies according to the citation style: Such as, in APA, it is the reference page, in MLA, it is the works referenced, and in Chicago A, it is the bibliography.

There are also variations in the sequence of information and how each entry is formatted. The format is frequently determined by the type of source (e.g. book, website, or journal article). A citation generator is the simplest approach to creating reference entries. Some citation styles additionally offer formatting guidelines for the entire article. This could contain formatting standards for the cover page, margins, spacing, font size, titles and headings, and even how to write numbers and abbreviations. These rules, on the other hand, are more flexible and less crucial than citation rules. Check to see whether your citation style provides formatting rules, but if it does not, then aim for a clear, consistent, and readable manner. Always check your university department's standards or the target journal's submission procedures beforehand to gain better insights.

Suggestions

User-friendly software for writing references:
- Zotero
- EndNote
- Mendeley
- Citations assist
- ReadCube
- Paperpile
- PaperDigest
- BibGuru
- Zbib.org
- EasyBib
- Cite this for me

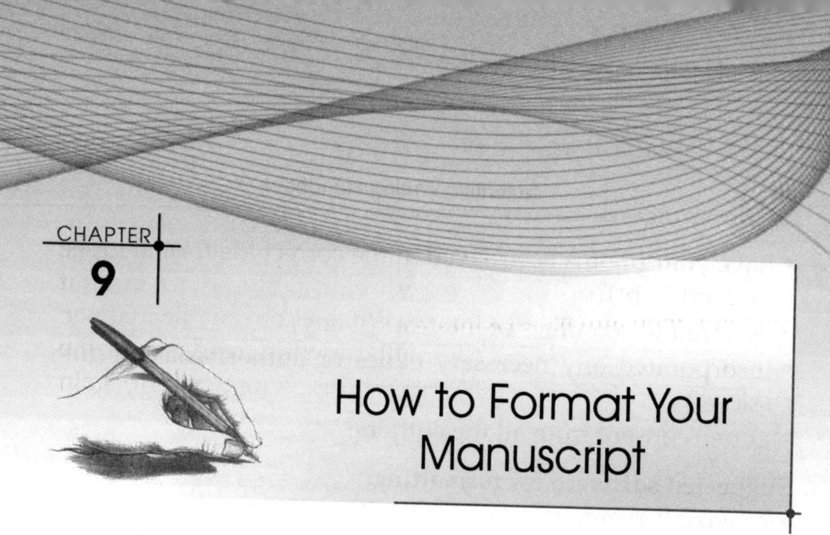

How to Format Your Manuscript

It is crucial to format your manuscript according to the requirements of the journal you want to submit it to, the details of which can be found in the instructions for authors of the respective journal's website. The submission process will be speed up because the journal's editorial team will not have to return your work to you for formatting. It can also assist you in succeeding because you will remember to supply any resources that the journal may demand.

TIP: Before completing a full draft of your work, it is a good idea to choose an initial target journal. After that, go to the journal's website and study the formatting rules before composing your draft. This might save you a lot of time, as you will not have to reformat an already-written article after selecting the journal!

Examine all the guidelines and make sure your manuscript complies with them. Also, you can use the below check list.

Have you ever:

- adhered to all word and character limits (title, running title, abstract, and manuscript text)?
- completed all of the sections that are required?
- completed the language requirements?
- provided all the contact information that was requested?
- are the figures in the correct location (in the text, at the end of the document, or in separate files)?
- is it possible to find references that have been properly formatted?

- have your photos been saved in the correct file format (.jpg,.png,.pdf,.ppt)?
- declared the conflicts of interest? (if any)
- incorporated any necessary ethics or authoritarian permissions?
- gotten consent from all the authors?

Suggested software for formatting:
- Microsoft Word
- Latex
- Overleaf

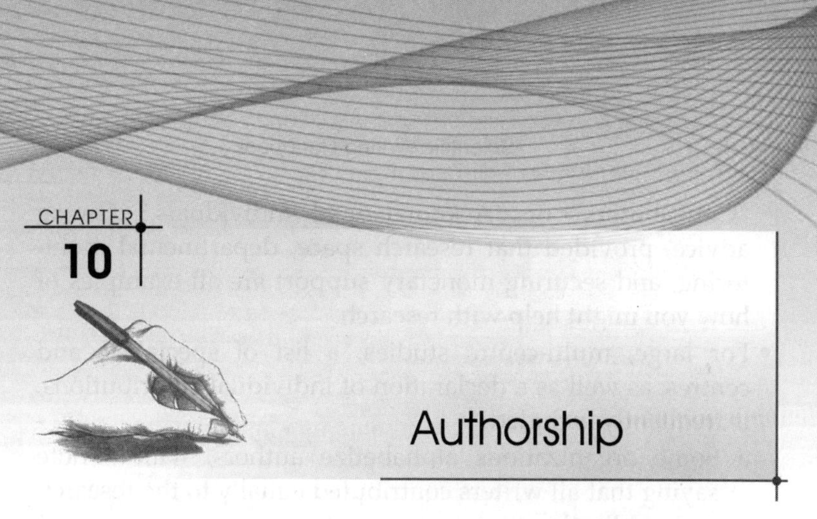

Authorship

The correct people gain credit for the effort and are held accountable for it when they are the authors of a scientific journal. Misrepresenting a scientist's connection to their work on purpose is considered a form of misconduct that erodes trust in the reporting of the work. While there is no universal definition of authorship, an "author" is usually believed to be someone who has made a major contribution to the intellectual substance of the work. "All persons identified as authors should qualify for authorship," according to the International Committee of Medical Journal Editors (ICMJE) guidelines for authorship.

The following criteria must all be met to be accredited as an author:

- Significantly aided in the idea and design of the study, as well as contributed to collecting data, analysis, and interpretation. For intellectual content, the article is being authored or amended.
- A person who has accepted the final version of the article.
- Acceptance of full responsibility for all areas of the work that involve the accuracy or integrity of any component.

The following are some broad standards that may vary per field:

- To determine authorship order, "a joint decision of the co-authors" should be employed.
- Individuals who take part in a study but do not match the journal's authorship requirements should be labelled

"Contributors" or "Acknowledged Individuals." Giving advice, provided that research space, departmental monitoring, and securing monetary support are all examples of how you might help with research.

- For large, multi-centre studies, a list of specialists and centres, as well as a declaration of individual contributions, is frequently included.

  a. Some organizations alphabetize authors, with a note saying that all writers contributed equally to the research and publication.

  b. "Ghost" authors, who make significant contributions but are not acknowledged or given authorship (for example, commercial sponsors);

  c. "Guest" authors, who make no discernible contributions but are listed just to increase the likelihood of publishing their research (example-senior of your university, department, or colleague); and "Gift" authors, whose contribution is based solely on a shaky affiliation with a study (examples—junior or senior of your department, colleague). These authorships are considered as unethical authorship.

- If they are not addressed properly, authorship conflicts may arise. Some arguments arise from misconduct (such as lying about one's role); others arise from interpretation concerns, such as the extent to which a person's contribution can be considered "important" and whether authorship is merited. Other issues could include being a participant in a study but not being identified as an author or collaborator; someone stealing your idea and writing a paper claiming full authorship; and your identity being published without your permission.

- If a disagreement is reported, an investigation may be launched with the journal editor and the author's institution to find a solution. Because ambiguity and misinterpretation are possible, it is strongly advised that a meeting be held before the research begins to document how each person would be acknowledged. Issues of authorship can be difficult and sensitive. When presented with such conditions, early-career academics may be scared that speaking up may jeopardize their reputation and career. In most cases, take the time to research each journal's authorship guidelines as well as industry standards.

Plagiarism and Copyright

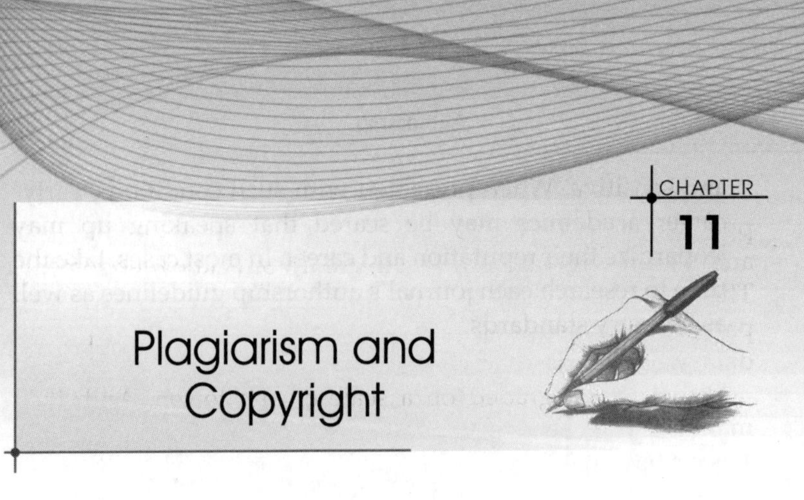

The act of portraying someone else's work as your own is known as plagiarism. When a writer plagiarises material on purpose, such as by copying and pasting or purchasing an essay from a website and submitting it as original work, is known as plagiarism. This frequently occurs because the individual has not handled his or her time well and has left the work to the last minute, or has battled with the writing process or topic. Any of these factors can drive a writer to desperation, causing them to steal someone else's ideas and claim credit for themself.

Journal editors and readers have a right to anticipate that submitted material is the author's original, that it has not been plagiarised (that is, copied without permission from other authors if permission is required), and that copyright has not been violated.

In other circumstances, a writer may plagiarise unintentionally owing to inattention, haste, or misunderstanding. For example, if bibliographical information is not recorded, a writer may be unable to produce a comprehensive and accurate citation. A writer might just copy and paste a piece from a website into the paper and then forget where he she got it. A procrastinating writer may speed through a draft, resulting in shoddy paraphrasing and erroneous quotations. Any of these behaviours could look to be plagiarised and result in undesirable consequences.

Hence, plagiarism is one of the most common types of publishing misconduct, where the author takes another's work and uses it without permission, credit, or acknowledgement. This can take several forms, ranging from direct copying to paraphrasing someone else's work, and can include either data, words, phrases or concepts and ideas.

Plagiarism is graded on a scale of one to ten. And, it is mandatory to check for the following:

- Is it a few lines, paragraphs, pages, or the complete piece that was taken?
- Is it the outcomes, the techniques, or the introduction that have been plagiarised?

Always remember that crediting the work of others is an important aspect of the process when it comes to your work. Position your work in the perspective of the field's growth and acknowledge the discoveries of others on which your research is based. Table 11.1 describes the commonly occurring unethical issues.

Follow these steps to avoid unintentional/accidental plagiarism:

- Recognize the different types of information that must be cited.
- Recognize what constitutes a source's fair dealing.
- Organize your source materials and notes carefully.
- Follow the summarizing, paraphrasing, and quoting require-ments.

Self-plagiarism

Refers to copying or using one's research work published already without citing the journal or book in which it has been published. This is mostly done by the authors to increase one's reputation. However, this is considered a serious violation of copy right when the author does not give due credit to the journal in which it has been published and is of much importance because once when the author submits their research work, the article becomes a part of the journal/book in which it has been published, this is the reason why every journal asks Copyright form or declaration form signed from

Table 11.1: Common unethical issues faced by the authors			
Action	**What is it?**	**Is it unethical?**	**What should you do?**
Literal copying	Not taking permission from the respective author or not acknowledging the source, reproducing a work and reproducing word by word in whole or in part.	Yes	Keep track of the sources you utilized during your study and where they appeared in your work.
Substantial copying	This can include research materials processes, tables or equipment	Yes	In your paper, make sure you fully credit and correctly cite the source.
Paraphrasing	Reproducing someone else's ideas while not copying word for word but rather using it without permission and acknowledging of the source	Yes	Keep a complete track of all the references used for your study. And ensure that you can comprehend what the original author is saying. So, never copy and paste words that you do not completely comprehend. Consider how the source's main concepts apply to your work until you can give the knowledge to others without mentioning the source.

Contd...

Table 11.1: Common unethical issues faced by the authors *(Contd.)*			
Action	**What is it?**	**Is it unethical?**	**What should you do?**
			Compare your paraphrasing to the original to ensure that the intended meaning is preserved, even if the words are changed.
Text-recycling	Reproducing parts of an author's work in a paper and submitting it for publication as a completely new article.	Yes	Put everything copied straight from a previously published paper in quotes, even if you are rephrasing it in your own words, make sure you cite the source correctly.

all its authors before publishing in their journal. However, it is to be noted that, self-citing can be done only in cases when the past research work published by one self is relevant to the present research.

Levels of plagiarism and the penalties

Plagiarism is a serious offence wherein one steals the work or ideas of another without giving due credit to the concerned author/authors. This could lead to severe penalties (as listed in Table 11.2), apart from failing exams or assignments and expulsion from the course as well for a student. On professional fronts, it can lead to spoiling one's reputation, loss of job, or result in legal action, especially if copyright infringement is involved. Hence, it is suggested to follow ethical guidelines to avoid these bitter consequences.

Table 11.2: Levels of plagiarism and its consequences			
Levels of plagiarism	**Severity of plagiarism**	**Penalties and Punishments**	
		For the thesis and dissertation (for students)	**For academic and research publication (for researcher and faculty)**
1	10 to 40%	Students should revise the manuscript and resubmit within the stipulated time, not exceeding 6 months	Will be asked to withdraw the manuscript
2	40 to 60%	Will be debarred from submitting a revised manuscript for one year.	• Will be asked to withdraw the submission • One annual increment will be denied. • Will not be allowed to function as a supervisor for students for 2 years
3	Above 60%	Cancellation of registration	• Will be asked to withdraw the submission • Two successive annual increments will be denied. • Will not be allowed to function as a supervisor for stud ents for 3 years

Contd...

Table 11.2: Levels of plagiarism and its consequences *(Contd.)*			
Levels of plagiarism	**Severity of plagiarism**	**Penalties and Punishments**	
		For the thesis and dissertation (for students)	**For academic and research publication (for researcher and faculty)**
Note 2	Penalty in cases where the benefit/ degree has been obtained already	Degree or credit will be suspended for a period recommended by IAIP and approved by the head of the concerned institution.	Benefit/credit will be made in abeyance for the period recommended by IAIP and approved by the head of the institution.

Framed by Institutional Academic Integrity Panel (IAIP)

Suggestions

Some Software/tools available for checking plagiarism are:
- Free software: DupliChecker, Copyleaks, PlagScan, Plagiarism checker, PaperRater, Paraphraser, BibMe, PlagTracker, Small SEQ tools, Unicheck, Quetext, Plagium, Search engine reports
- Paid software: iThenticate, Turnitin, Grammarly, Copy Scape, Viper (scan my essay) PlagAware, Urkund and Oxsico

Research Fraud

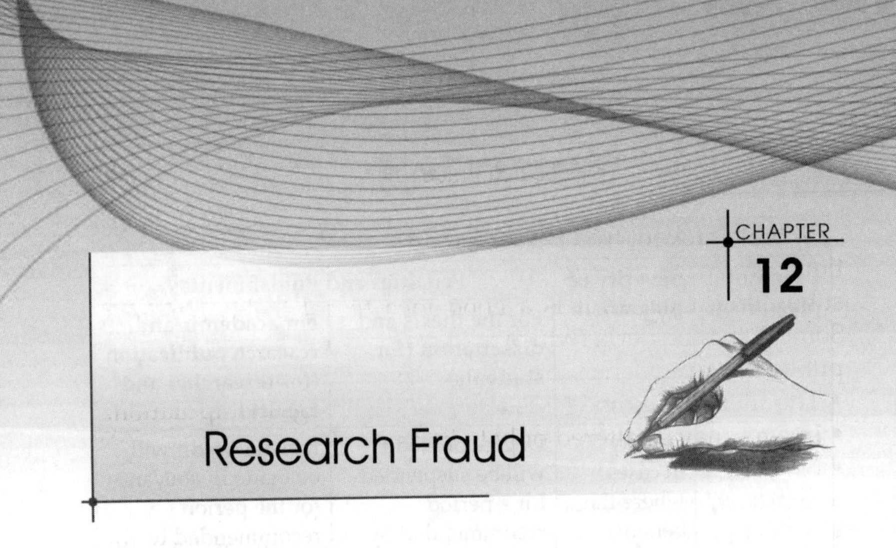

Research fraud is defined as the act of publishing data or conclusions that were not derived from tests or observations, but rather through invention or data manipulation. There are two categories of research and scientific publishing:

1. *Fabrication:* Creating and recording research data and results which have never been carried out during the entire research but presented in a manner just to make it consistent with similar articles is called fabrication. Also called "cooked up."

2. *Falsification:* Manipulation of study materials, photographs, data, equipment, or processes. When data or results are changed or withheld in such a way that the research is not fairly portrayed, this is referred to as falsification. A person may fabricate data to achieve the intended result of making the study significant.

Fabrication and falsification are both instances of scientific misconduct that result in a scientific record that does not accurately reflect observable truth.

Certain instances of fraud are easy to spot, such as when a referee knows for a fact that a given laboratory lacks the requisite equipment to conduct the reported research. If an image looks to have been altered or is a combination of several different tests. The control experiment results may be "too perfect." In such circumstances, an investigation would be conducted to determine whether a fraud had occurred.

To help prevent fraud, most publishers include strict restrictions on image change and access to reported data. Before submitting a paper, it is a good idea to get to know them. Some general criteria (which may range from field to field and publisher to publisher) are as follows:

- The alteration of images is referred to as image manipulation.
- Images may be altered only to improve clarity.
- No single feature can be improved, hidden, relocated, removed, or introduced within an image.
- Adjustments to brightness, contrast, and colour balance are usually allowed as long as they do not conceal or delete any information from the original.
- When submitting an article for editorial review, authors may be asked to supply raw data. As a result, all data for a particular study should be kept for a reasonable period following publication. The data should have a designated custodian.
- Human studies, such as clinical trials, have strict requirements for data retention length.

Common ethical problems which occur while writing research have been in Table 12.1:

Table 12.1: Unethical practices with data		
Action	**Possible ethical issues**	**What should you not do?**
Data that has been intentionally modified, changed, or omitted.	Never tamper with or modify data. Keep meticulous records of your information. Raw data records should be available in case an editor requests them, even if your research has already been published. Learn about the publisher's data rules before submitting an article.	Manipulating data
Includes the materials, methodologies,	Make sure you know what you're permitted to do with an image to improve clarity	Manipulating data images

Contd...

Table 12.1: Unethical practices with data *(Contd.)*		
Action	**Possible ethical issues**	**What should you not do?**
tables, and equipment utilized in research.	before submitting your work. Even if you believe the image changes are permissible, you should notify the journal before submitting your work. Compare any data images used to support your work to the original image data to ensure that no changes have been made.	

Hence, unethical practices such as fabrication and falsification must be strictly avoided, failing to which can invite serious consequences.

Ethics in Scientific Research and Publication

To a large part, academic publishing is built on trust. Editors have faith in peer reviewers to make fair assessments, authors have faith in editors to choose qualified peer reviewers, and readers have faith in the peer-review process. Academic publishing also takes place in a world where significant intellectual, financial, and occasionally political interests conflict or compete. Academic societies, journal editors, authors, research funders, readers, and publishers will all benefit from sound judgments and effective editorial processes designed to handle these competing interests.

Important Checklist

Who funded the project?

Readers have a right to know who paid for a research endeavour or a document's publishing. All research publications should include a list of research funders. Any funding for a publication, whether from a commercial enterprise, a charity, or a government agency, should be stated clearly in the publication. This is true for any type of paper (including, for example, research papers, review papers, letters, editorials, commentaries).

What was the source of the labour?

The list of authors should reflect the ones who completed the work correctly. One or more writers should be given credit for all published work. The notions of academic authorship should be explained to writers in the journal instructions, as well as which contributions qualify for authorship and which do not.

Authorship rules [for example, the International Committee of Medical Journal Editors (ICMJE) requirements] should be reminded of contributors, and suitable authorship disclosures should be used to encourage their adherence.

Editors should request a declaration confirming all authors meet the journal's authorship standards and that no one who meets these criteria has been left off the list.

Editors should get a statement from the authors stating that they have acknowledged all major contributions to their publication made by individuals who did not match the journal's authorship criteria. Author editors, statisticians, medical writers, and translators, for example, may be included, depending on their contribution.

If an authorship disagreement or discrepancy arises before publication (for example, after submission, modifications to the list of authors are proposed), editors should take care to explain the situation.

Individual contributions to the research and publication process are listed, which provides more transparency than traditional authorship lists and may deter unethical authorship practices such as 'ghost' authors those who qualify for authorship but are not listed and 'guest' or honorary authors, individuals who are listed despite not qualifying for authorship, such as heads of department not directly involved with research.

If an authorship dispute arises after publication (for example, if someone contacts the editor claiming they should have been an author of a published paper or requesting that their name be removed from a paper), the editor should contact the corresponding author and, if possible, the other authors to verify the case's veracity. Genuine errors are unlikely if authorship policies have been properly defined and an explicit authorship declaration(s) has been received.

Most journals only want to publish work that has never been published before. One reason for this is that duplicate publication might influence the scientific literature, which can have serious repercussions, such as when results are unintentionally included in meta-analyses multiple times. Both journal editors and readers have a right to know if a study has been published before.

If a main research report is published and later discovered to be redundant (that is, it has already been published), the editor should contact the authors and consider publishing a redundant publication notice. Editors have the right to require original work and ask writers about whether opinion pieces (for example, editorials, letters, and non-systematic reviews) have previously been published; journals should create a guideline on how much overlap between such publications is acceptable.

Papers that present new analyses or syntheses of previously published data (for example, sub-group analyses) should include a reference to the primary data source, including a reference to the clinical trial registration number if one is available and a complete reference to the related primary publications.

Journals that publish clinical trials should think about making registration a prerequisite for publishing. Even if a journal does not require clinical trial registration before publishing, editors should encourage unambiguous identification of clinical trials and have a strategy in place for how such information is presented within the final article's structure. If editors suspect research misconduct (such as data fabrication, falsification, or plagiarism), they should make every effort to have the matter thoroughly investigated by the right authorities. Peer review can occasionally disclose suspicions of wrongdoing. Editors should make sure that peer reviewers are aware of this potential function. Serious misconduct (for example, data fabrication, falsification, incorrect picture modification, or plagiarism) should be treated seriously by peer reviewers. Authors, on the other hand, have the right to react to such charges and for investigations to be conducted in a timely and thorough manner. Although journals are rarely in a position to investigate complaints of wrongdoing, editors have a responsibility to notify appropriate entities (for example, employers, sponsors, and regulatory authorities) and encourage them to do so.

Editors should establish publication policies that encourage ethical and responsible research. Editors should verify that studies have been approved by appropriate authorities (for example, Institutional Review Board, research ethics committee, data and safety monitoring board, and regulatory authorities including those overseeing animal experiments). Peer reviewers should be encouraged by editors to think about ethical issues posed by the research they are examining. If editors believe it is necessary, they should ask authors for additional information.

When individual human subjects or case studies are discussed (for example, in medicine, psychology, or criminology), journals should maintain confidentiality and not publish information that could upset or harm participants/subjects, or compromise the confidentiality of, say the doctor–patient relationship. If there have been ethical violations, editors should inform readers. General advice on retractions has been published by Blackwell Publishing. If work is confirmed to be fraudulent, journals should 'publish retractions,' or 'expressions of concern,' if editors have reasonable suspicions of misconduct.

Conflict of Interest

Editors, authors, and peer reviewers must disclose any potential conflicts of interest that might impair their ability to present or review data fairly. Examples: Personal, political, intellectual, religious interests or financial.

Journal editors have a responsibility to guarantee that the information they publish is accurate. Authors and readers should be encouraged to notify journals if they find flaws in published material. If inaccuracies are identified that potentially impact the interpretation of data or information offered in an article, editors should post revisions. Retractions and statements of concern about misbehaviour should be distinguished from corrections resulting from flaws within a publication by authors or journals.

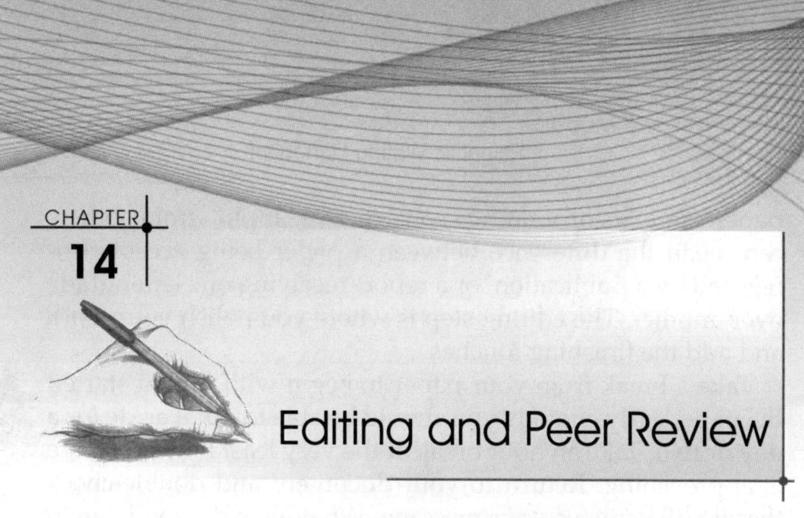

Editing and Peer Review

A journal editor typically screens a manuscript once it is submitted to a journal and determines whether to send it for full peer review. After passing the initial screening, a manuscript is sent to one or more peer reviewers. For journal publication, there are three forms of peer review:

- The names of reviewers are not divulged to the writers in a single-blind review.
- The names of the reviewers and authors are kept hidden from each other in a double-blinded review.
- The names of writers and reviewers are revealed to each other in an open peer review process.

Finally, the peer reviewers' reports are considered by journal editors or the editorial board, who make the final decision on whether to approve or reject the paper for publication. Peer review is essentially a quality control technique for journal publication. It is a procedure in which specialists assess scholarly works to ensure that published science is of high quality and also as per the journal guidelines/standards. Peer reviewers, on the other hand, do not make the final decision on whether to accept or reject publications. They can just provide a recommendation. Journal editors or the journal's editorial board have sole decision-making authority in peer-reviewed journals. Indeed, the journal editor is seen as a key player in the decision-making process.

You are not finished yet, even though you have finished collecting data and drafting your report. Re-reading your paper and incorporating constructive input from others can mean the difference between a paper being accepted or rejected by a publication, or a report receiving one letter grade over another. The editing step is where you polish your work and add the finishing touches.

Take a break from your paper to begin with. If you started the paper early enough, you should be able to put it aside for a day or two. Take an hour break at the very least if the deadline is approaching. Return to your document and double-check that it still conveys your message. What gaps do you have in your tale structure? What has not been thoroughly explained? Where does your writing become clumsy, making it harder to follow your point? Consider reading the article aloud first, then printing and editing a hard copy to examine it from several perspectives.

Make sure you addressed all the study's primary topics on the first pass through your work. One approach to accomplish this is to jot down the main themes you wish to cover before re-reading your paper. You may need to eliminate several paragraphs if your paper deviates from these topics. If you forget to include something, on the other hand, include it. Check the flow of your paragraphs by making sure that each paragraph has a common thread connecting it to the one before it, and that each sentence inside a paragraph builds on the one before it. A classmate is good because he or she is familiar with the assignment and could help you exchange papers. When editing someone else's paper, follow the same methods indicated above. If you cannot find a classmate, ask a family member or a friend. Having a fresh pair of eyes look at your work can help you spot areas of your paper that need to be clarified. This technique will also provide you with insight into the peer review process, which is an important part of professional science writing. Negative remarks should not discourage you; incorporating reviewer criticism can only strengthen your paper. It is constructive to receive constructive criticism.

Peer reviewers make an independent recommendation to the journal editor about whether the paper should be accepted or rejected (with or without revisions). The journal editor weighs all of the criticism received from peer reviewers before deciding whether to accept or reject the paper. Peer review is the method by which journals examine and regulate the quality of the information they publish by allowing experts in the field to review and comment on articles that have been submitted. And first screening of manuscripts submitted to a journal is performed by the editorial team. Those who pass the screening receive peer evaluation from at least two specialists. Peer reviewers make an independent recommendation to the journal editor about whether the paper should be accepted or rejected (with or without revisions).

Top journals are frequently obliged to reject even high-quality manuscripts due to a huge number of submissions or a lack of match with the journal's editorial focus due to a big number of submissions. While reviewers and editors may easily agree on what should not be published, selecting what is worthy of publication is a more difficult task. Finally, journal editors make decisions on whether or not to accept or reject papers based on their assessment of the papers' publishing potential and feedback from reviewers.

Writing a Systematic Review

What is a systematic review?

A "high-level review of primary research on a certain topic," based on high-quality research shreds of evidence published previously.

The phases of writing a systematic review are:

- Identifying
- Selecting/screening
- Synthesizing/eligibility
- Appraisal/finalizing/including

A systematic review is a research study that aims to gather and analyze all available data from multiple studies on the same topic to address a specific research question comprehensively. Before beginning the systematic review, the authors establish criteria for choosing which evidence should be included or eliminated. This reduces the danger of bias and improves the reliability of the results.

Systematic reviews should:

- Declare objectives with an explicit and repeatable approach.
- Use a rigorous search strategy to find all studies that match the eligibility requirements.
- Assess the validity of the findings of the included studies; and
- Synthesize the findings of the studies in a systematic manner.

Steps for writing a systematic review

Writing a systematic review is rigorous but worthy since this type of research stands as the most valuable research. This is a more structured process and requires careful planning, and precision in executing the methodologies apart from ensuring reliability to the work. Flowchart 15.1 serves as a road map to navigate through this process

1. Formulate a research question

Before you begin your project, consider whether a systematic review is required. Is there a book on your subject that has previously been written? Librarians can assist you in your search. Determine whether you have adequate time and resources to perform a thorough evaluation. Keep in mind that finishing it could take more than a year. Form a team of collaborators to assist you. This lowers the chance of prejudice.

Put your issue into the *"Well-Built Clinical Question"* framework to start your systematic review.

PICO (population, intervention, comparison and outcomes) stands for four basic aspects, and your query should address them all. PICO is used for quantitative articles and is a vital component in a systematic review.

2. Develop research protocol

A research protocol is a step-by-step method for investigating a biological or health-related problem. Details such as these should be included in systematic review protocols (objectives of your project should):

a. specify the methodologies and processes to be used;

b. include the eligibility criteria for individual studies (such as research design);

c. project how data from individual studies will be extracted; and

d. what analysis will be conducted?

Consider using *PROSPERO* to register your review protocol for free. *PROSPERO* allows reviews with health-related outcomes, such as those on the following topics:

• health and social care,

• welfare,

Flowchart 15.1: PRISMA flow diagram

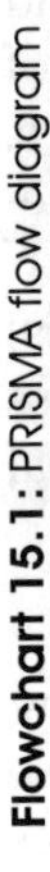

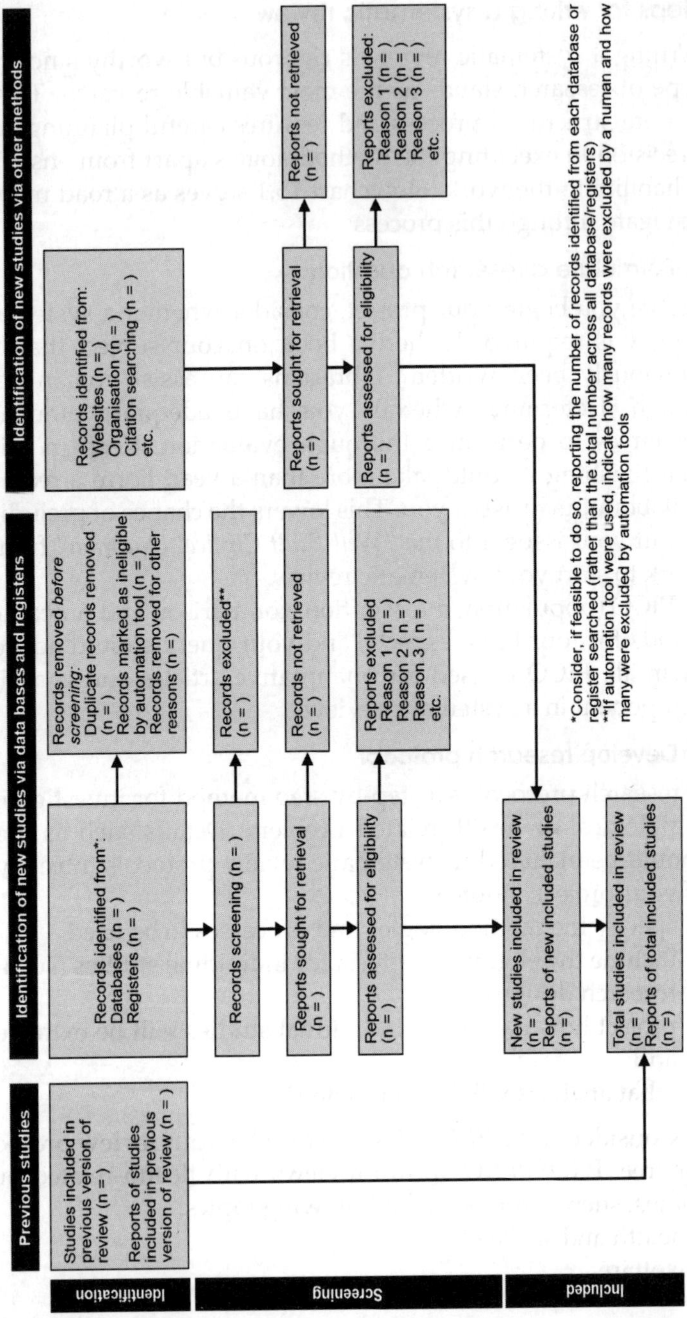

Source: PRISMA statement.org

- education,
- public health,
- international development and
- crime and justice

3. Conduct literature search

When planning your search strategy, the Institute of Medicine suggests collaborating with a librarian. Your goal is to locate all relevant papers on your issue, therefore, do a thorough literature search. A librarian will assist you in selecting databases that are relevant to your topic and developing a comprehensive search strategy. You should also go outside of the traditional academic publishing model. "Grey literature" is a term used to describe this type of writing. Searching conference proceedings, visiting pharmaceutical company websites, and contacting specialists in the field are all possibilities. Negative results are less likely to be published, hence the grey literature is significant. This will have an impact on the accuracy of your results.

Always, keep detailed records as you search and document details such as:
- the databases you searched and the years they covered;
- the dates the searches were initially performed and updated;
- the techniques you employed, including search phrases; and
- the number of results you got.

You can also use a *citation manager*. These tools can create bibliographies, remove duplicate records, and share citations with a team.

4. Select studies as per the protocol

Two reviewers should be assigned to the task of screening studies. Make use of the criteria listed in your protocol. Titles and abstracts can be used for the first round of screening. The full-text publications for selected research should be reviewed in a second round of screening. Reviewers should maintain track of studies that were excluded, as well as the reason for their exclusion.

5. Appraise studies per protocol

At least two reviewers should assess the methodological soundness of a sample of full-text articles. Use a checklist to see if the studies match the protocol's requirements. Questions to address include:

a. were the patients randomly assigned to groups?
b. was the allocation sequence hidden from patients and doctors?
c. could the study's conclusions have been influenced by bias?

6. Extract data

Make a form for extracting data. At least two reviewers should be assigned to extract data from the included research. Researchers can customize Cochrane's templates for their projects.

7. Analyze results

Make a table of study findings and, if applicable, a forest plot to show the relative strength of treatment effects. Analyze data for concerns like heterogeneity (differences between studies) and sensitivity of findings. Consider conducting a meta-analysis of the findings. Also, facilitate access to excluded research for readers who are interested.

8. Interpret results

Limitations (including biases), evidence strength, applicability, economic consequences, and implications for future practice or study should all be considered. The *Cochrane Handbook* gives thorough instructions on how to interpret findings and develop conclusions.

PRISMA (Preferred Reporting Items for Systematic Reviews and Meta-Analysis) is a 27-item checklist (Table 15.1) used for reporting systematic reviews and meta-analysis. This checklist serves as an instant guide for the researchers as this serves to maintain transparency in publishing.

Table 15.1: PRISMA check list for researcher		
Section/topic	**S. no**	**Checklist item**
TITLE		
Title	1	Find out if the report is a systematic review
ABSTRACT		
Structured summary	2	Should include the following essential headings, namely, a. Title: Identify if the report is a systematic review. b. Background: Provide the objectives of the review. c. Methods: Specify the inclusion and exclusion criteria, data sources with the date on which the last data was searched, including the methods used for assessing the bias of the studies included for this review, study appraisal and synthesis methodologies. d. Results: Include the total number of studies included along with the details of the participants and summarise the relevant characteristics of the studies, mention the results of the main outcome by including the number of studies and the number of participants for each of these. e. Discussion: Include the limitations in terms of risk of bias, inconsistency, and imprecision. Interpret the results and include the important implications. f. Other: Mention the primary source of funding, and systematic review registration number.

Contd.

Table 15.1: PRISMA check list for researcher *(Contd.)*		
Section/topic	**S. no**	**Checklist item**
INTRODUCTION		
Rationale	3	Explain why the review is necessary considering what is previously known.
Objectives	4	Provide a clear summary of the topics that will be addressed, including Participants, Interventions, Comparisons, Outcomes, and Study methodology (PICOS).
METHODS		
Eligibility criteria	5	Mention the reason for inclusion and exclusion criteria and how the studies were grouped for the analysis.
Information sources	6	Describe all the information sources employed during the search along with the date last searched (e.g. websites, registers, organisations, reference lists)
Search strategy	7	Present a complete electronic search strategy used, including any limits that were utilised, so that it may be replicated. Include the list of filters and limits employed.
Study selection process	8	Describe the method for picking studies (i.e. screening, eligibility, included in a systematic review, and, if applicable, included in the meta-analysis). Include the number of reviewers involved in the screening of each report and if they worked independently. Also, mention the automation tools used (if any).
Data collection process	9	Describe the mechanism for extracting data from reports (e.g. piloted forms, separately, in duplicate) as well as any procedures for receiving and confirming information from investigators and if the investigators reviewed each report independently.

Contd.

Table 15.1: PRISMA check list for researcher *(Contd.)*		
Section/topic	**S. no**	**Checklist item**
Data items	10a	List and specify all the outcomes for which data was taken. Please indicate whether the researchers actively sought all the results aligned with the defined outcome domains in each study, including various measures, time points, and analytical approaches. If not, describe the criteria and methods employed to determine which results were prioritized for collection.
	10b	Enumerate and provide explanations for all additional variables for which data were sought (such as participant and intervention attributes, and funding sources). Also, elucidate any inferences or assumptions made when encountering data that was either missing or unclear.
Risk of bias in individual studies	11	Outline the methods used to assess bias risk in the included studies, including the tools, number of reviewers, their independence, and any automation tools. Describe how this assessment, whether at the study or outcome level, will inform data synthesis.
Summary measures	12	List the most important summary measures (e.g. risk ratio, difference in means).
Synthesis of results	13a	For each meta-analysis, describe the methodology for managing data and merging study results, if applicable, including measures of consistency.
	13b	Explain any necessary steps to prepare the data for presentation or synthesis, like addressing missing summary statistics or performing data conversions.

Contd.

Table 15.1: PRISMA check list for researcher *(Contd.)*

Section/topic	S. no	Checklist item
	13c	Describe the methods used for tabulating or displaying the results of individual studies and syntheses visually.
	13d	Enumerate the methods used for synthesizing the results and provide a rationale for the choices.
	13e	Explain the methods used to identify the possible causes of heterogeneity among study results (e.g. subgroup analysis, meta-regression).
	13f	Specify if sensitivity analyses were performed to gauge the robustness of the aggregated findings
Reporting of risk of bias across studies	14	Specify any assessment of risk of bias that may affect the cumulative evidence (e.g. publication bias, selective reporting within studies).
Assessment of certainty	15	Detail the techniques used to gauge the level of confidence or certainty in the evidence related to a specific outcome.
RESULTS		
Study selection	16a	Give the number of studies that were screened, evaluated for eligibility, and included in the review, as well as the reasons for exclusions at each stage, preferably in the form of a flow diagram.
	16b	Provide citations for studies which meet the inclusion criteria and the details of which were excluded and why.
Study characteristics	17	Provide citations for each study and the features for which data were retrieved (e.g. study size, PICOS, follow-up time).

Contd.

Table 15.1: PRISMA check list for researcher *(Contd.)*		
Section/topic	**S. no**	**Checklist item**
Risk of bias within studies	18	Provide information on each study's risk of bias and, if available, any result-level assessments.
Results of individual studies	19	For all outcomes, provide, for each study: (a) Relevant summary statistics for each group, as applicable, and (b) an effect estimate along with its confidence intervals, preferably presented in structured tables or forest plots.
Synthesis of results	20a	For each synthesis, provide a concise summary of the contributing studies' characteristics and their risk of bias.
	20b	Display the outcomes of all statistical syntheses performed. If a meta-analysis was conducted, present the summary estimate, its precision (e.g. confidence/credible interval), and measures of statistical heterogeneity for each analysis. When comparing groups, elucidate the direction of the effect.
	20c	Share the findings from all examinations of potential sources of heterogeneity among the study results.
	20d	Report the outcomes of all sensitivity analyses performed to evaluate the resilience of the combined results.
Risk of bias across studies	21	Present results of any assessment of the risk of bias across studies occurring due to reporting bias for every synthesis assessed.
Certainty of evidence	22	Provide evaluations of the level of certainty (or confidence) in the body of evidence for each assessed outcome.

Contd.

Table 15.1: PRISMA check list for researcher *(Contd.)*		
Section/topic	**S. no**	**Checklist item**
DISCUSSION		
Summary of evidence	23a	Offer a broad interpretation of the findings concerning existing evidence and context.
	23b	Examine and address the constraints or drawbacks of the evidence included in the review.
	23c	Address any review process limitations.
	23d	Explore the implications of the results for practice, policy, and future research
OTHER INFORMATION		
Registration and protocol	24a	Furnish registration details for the review, specifying the register name and registration number, or declare if the review was not registered.
	24b	Specify the location where the review protocol is accessible, or mention if a protocol was not created.
	24c	Elaborate and clarify any changes or revisions made to the information initially presented during registration or in the review protocol.
Support	25	Detail the origins of financial or non-financial support for the review, and elucidate the role of the funders or sponsors in the review process.
Competing interests	26	Declare any potential conflicts of interest involving the authors who conducted the review.
Accessibility of data, code, and other materials	27	State which of the following are publicly accessible and provide their locations: template data collection forms, data extracted from included studies, data used for all analyses, analytic code, and any other materials utilized in the review.

Suggested Reading

PRISMA transparent reporting of systematic reviews and meta-analyses (for fetching details on PRISMA guidelines (abstract, expanded checklist, checklist)—2020.

Writing Meta-analysis

What is a meta-analysis?

A meta-analysis is a statistical analysis that combines the findings of two or more research. This term was coined by "Gene V Glass Symbol in the year 1976. Meta-analysis is yet another strong type of research design like that of systematic review.

Definitions by various authors:

- "An exercise in mega-silliness!" — Eyesnack, 1978.
- "A new bete noire (which represents) the unacceptable face of statics (and) should be stifled at birth" — Oakes, 1986.
- "Meta-analysis, Shmeta-analysis."— Shapiro, 1994.

Key points

- Meta-analyses may provide benefits such as increased precision, the ability to answer problems not addressed by individual studies, and the ability to resolve disagreements arising from competing claims. However, if specific study designs, within-study biases, variance among studies, and reporting biases are not carefully evaluated, they have the potential to mislead substantially.
- It is critical to understand the types of data (such as dichotomous and continuous) that result from measuring an outcome in a single research and to select appropriate effect measures for comparing intervention groups.
- Most meta-analysis approaches rely on a weighted average of the effect estimates from various studies.

- Studies that do not include any occurrences provide no information regarding the risk or odds ratio. *The Peto technique* is less biased and more powerful than other methods for unusual events.
- Variation between studies (heterogeneity) must be considered, even though most Cochrane Reviews lack sufficient data to allow for a reliable analysis of its causes. By assuming that underlying effects follow a normal distribution, random-effects meta-analyses allow for heterogeneity, but they must be evaluated cautiously.
- Prediction intervals from random-effects meta-analyses are a valuable tool for displaying the degree of variation between studies. To prepare a meta-analysis, many decisions must be made. To see if general findings are resilient to potentially influential decisions, sensitivity analysis should be utilized.

The critical examination of whether it is suitable to combine the numerical data of all, or possibly some, of the research is a key stage in a systematic review. In a meta-analysis, a statistical measure, along with its confidence interval, is generated to provide an overview of how effective an experimental intervention is when compared to a control or comparator intervention.

Some of the potential benefits of meta-analysis are as follows:

1. To increase precision. Many studies are too small to give conclusive data about the impact of interventions on their own. Estimation is frequently enhanced when more data is available.
2. To provide answers to questions that were not addressed in the individual research. A specified type of participant and clearly defined interventions are common in primary research. A group of studies with different characteristics can be used to look into the consistency of effect over a broader variety of people and interventions. It may also enable the investigation of reasons for variations in effect estimates, if applicable.
3. To resolve conflicts that arise from seemingly contradictory studies or to propose new hypotheses. The degree of conflict

can be officially examined, and the causes for various results can be studied and quantified using a statistical synthesis of findings.

4. Of course, using statistical synthesis methods does not ensure the validity of a review's findings, just as it does not guarantee the validity of a main study's findings. Furthermore, statistical approaches, like any tool, can be abused.

Principles of meta-analysis

The main assumptions of meta-analysis are as follows.

Meta-analysis is usually divided into two stages, namely:

1. The first stage involves calculating a summary statistic for each research to describe the observed intervention effect in a consistent manner across all studies. If the data is dichotomous, the summary statistic might be a risk ratio, or if the data is continuous, it might be a difference between means.

2. In the second stage, a weighted average of the intervention effects reported in the various studies is calculated to produce a summary (combined) intervention effect estimate. The following is the definition of a weighted average:

   Where Yi is the intervention effect estimated in the ith study, Wi is the weight given to the ith study, and the summation is across all studies. The weighted average is equal to the mean intervention effect if all the weights are the same. The more weight the study is given, the more it contributes to the weighted average.

   a. The assumption that the studies are not all assessing the same intervention effect, but rather estimate intervention effects that follow a distribution across studies, might be included in the combination of intervention effect estimates across studies. A random-effects meta-analysis is built on this foundation. A fixed-effect meta-analysis, on the other hand, is undertaken if it is considered that each study is estimating the same quantity.

   b. The standard error of the summary intervention effect can be used to derive a confidence interval, which communicates the precision (or uncertainty) of the summary estimate; and to derive a P value, which comm-unicates the strength of the evidence against the null hypothesis of no intervention effect.

3. All meta-analysis methods can include an assessment of whether the variation among the results of the separate studies is compatible with random variation, or whether it is large enough to indicate inconsistency of intervention effects across studies, in addition to yielding a summary quantification of the intervention effect.

4. One of the many practical factors that must be considered while conducting a meta-analysis is the issue of missing data. Review authors should think about the consequences of missing participant outcome data, in particular.

Hence, perform a comprehensive literature search within databases. After you have settled on the PICO, you will do a literature search in the databases. This will assist you in determining the most appropriate search phrases. These search phrases are organized utilizing Boolean logic, fuzzy logic, particular search-related restricted language, truncation and expansion symbols, and positioning of the terms in different portions of a given study. The connectors "And," "Or," and "Not" are used in various combinations in Boolean Logic to expand or filter down search results and findings.

You can also use "fuzzy logic" to search for specific articles in addition to Boolean logic. When you utilize fuzzy logic, you search for highly particular articles using search keywords like "Adults" Near "Mindfulness" or "Adults "Within 5 Words of "Mindfulness." These can be mixed and matched in a variety of ways. Many databases, such as Pubmed/Medline, use MeSH (Medical Subject Headings) as a controlled vocabulary in which the database curators keep track of or archive different articles based on certain search criteria.

Ultimately, search terms can be found in various sections and components of a study report. Most studies' titles and abstracts can be used to search. Another area to look for information is in the body of the article. As a result of combining these tactics, you may conduct a thorough search of articles or research that will contain data for your meta-analysis. By reviewing the titles, abstracts, and full texts of the papers, you can choose which ones to use for meta-analysis.

To begin, study the titles and abstracts of all relevant papers that you come across during your search. But first, come up with a technique for selecting and rejecting publications for your meta-analysis. For instance, you can create a scheme in which you can write:

- The article is unrelated to the research question.
- The relevant population is missing from the article.
- The article lacks a relevant intervention (or exposure)
- The article lacks a relevant comparison group
- The article does not discuss the result of interest in this study
- The paper is presented in a non-standard style and is not suitable for review
- The article is published in a foreign language that cannot be translated
- The piece is published beyond the date ranges
- The article is a duplicate of another article

Use this method to go over every article you initially retrieved based on their titles and abstracts. Typically, simply one clause is sufficient to reject a study and mention that the study was rejected on that criterion, with the first clause being noted as the primary cause. So, even if a study can be rejected on two grounds, the first one is indicated as the major ground for rejection; you will need to create a process diagram to show which articles were rejected and why. PRISMA charts are a type of process diagram (Fig. 15.1).

After you have completed this stage and determined a particular number of studies that must be included in the meta-analysis, get the full texts of those studies. Then read the entire paragraph again and repeat the rejection exercise, noting the numbers. This round, you will reject fewer articles, as you might imagine. Then, to broaden your research read the complete text of these papers and hand search the reference lists. This is a crucial stage. Often, in this stage, you will discover sources that you will need to search for or writers whose work you will need to study to compile a comprehensive list of all works and research on the subject. This is an important step that should not be skipped. You will notice that several authors and research groups appear frequently in this stage; make a note of them; you may need to contact a few writers to see if they have published any additional research. All of these are required to conduct a thorough search of the research so that no studies that may be relevant to this meta-analysis are overlooked.

At the very least, you will need to figure out the following:

- What is the theory and theories that this study is based on?
- Does the sample size meet the research question's requirements? Is this investigation underpowered?
- Did the authors go to great lengths to eliminate biases in the study?
- Was there blinding, even if it was an RCT?
- What level of assurance do you have that the authors used a proper randomization procedure? What are the chances that the groups being compared were extremely different in terms of prognosis?
- Did the authors undertake an intention to treat analysis if this is an RCT?
- How did the authors avoid the possibility of selection bias in this observational study?
- How much was the risk of information bias from the participants eliminated?
- What confounding variables were controlled for? Are these confounding variables sufficient?

Strengths of Meta-analysis

- Imposes discipline
- Makes process explicit and systematic
- An organized way of combining a lot of information
- More differentiated and sophisticated than traditional reviews
- Combining studies increases the power
- Find 'significant' results

Weaknesses of Meta-analysis

- Biases—missing studies
- Heterogeneity—"apples and oranges"
- Can differ from previously published research (publication bias)
- GIGO ('Quality of Studies')—Garbage In and Garbage Out
- What is the definition of quality?
- Requires a lot of effort and subject-matter experience
- Statistic—mechanics may obfuscate theory
- Only useful for closed-ended problems

Abstract the data

- Multiple outcomes per study—multiple measurement points per outcome—Sub-samples per study population—meta-analytic data is naturally hierarchical
- Analysis usually invariably consists of a subset of coded effect sizes, resulting in many effect sizes per research. Those subsets must be able to be selected and created thanks to the data structure.
- To ensure statistical independence, each study can only have one effect size (or one effect size per sub-sample within a study).

To conclude, while the fundamentals of writing are usually taught early in childhood, many people try to improve their writing skills throughout their lives. Even professional scientists believe that they can always improve their writing skills. Focusing on the success techniques outlined in this article will improve your writing skills while also making the scientific writing process easier and more efficient. Keep in mind that, there is no one-size-fits-all is-all approach in writing a scientific paper, and as you acquire experience, you will begin to develop your style.

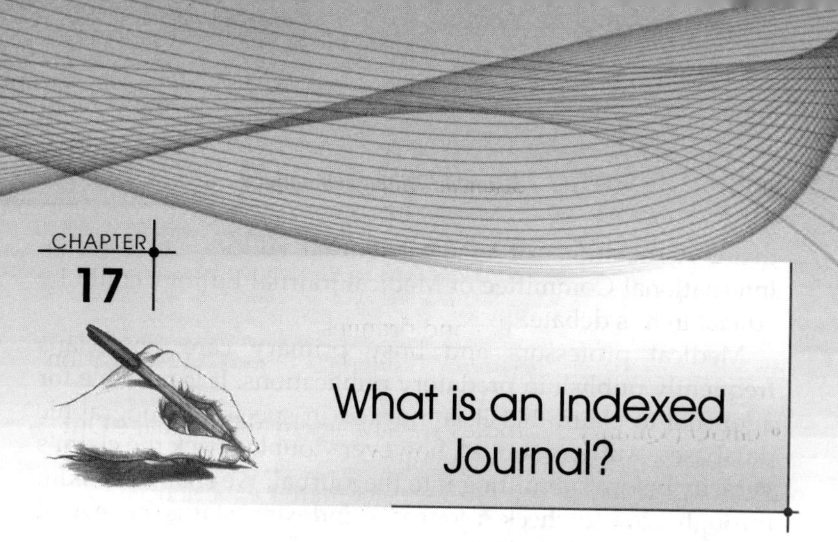

What is an Indexed Journal?

A journal's indexation is seen to be a reflection of its quality. In comparison to non-indexed publications, indexed journals are thought to be of greater scientific quality. Medical journal indexing has become a contentious topic. Index Medicus has long been regarded as the most comprehensive index of medical scientific journal publications. It has been in print since 1879. Many more prominent indexing systems have emerged throughout time. MedLine, PubMed, EMBASE, SCOPUS, EBSCO Publishing's Electronic Databases, and SCIRUS are only a few of them. Index Medicus is available in a variety of regional and national editions, including African Index Medicus.

Teaching faculty at medical colleges should also have indexed publications, according to MCI requirements. As a result, many more authors would be able to publish than ever before. Since there is no clarity on the topic, choosing a high-quality publication becomes a challenging decision for the authors. Should only journals indexed in Index Medicus/MedLine/PubMed be targeted? Is it acceptable to submit to journals with a high impact factor even if they are not indexed by Index Medicus/MedLine/PubMed?

Many more indexing services have recently emerged. Casper, DOAJ, Expanded Academic ASAP, Genamics Journal Seek, Hinari, Index Copernicus, Open J Gate, Primo Central, Pro Quest, SCOLOAR, SIIC databases, Summon by Serial Solutions, Ulrich's International Periodical Directory, and Ulrich's International Periodical Directory are among them. Associations of medical journal editors, such as the International Committee of Medical Journal Editors, could be crucial in this debate.

Medical professors and busy primary care physicians frequently publish in predatory publications. It is possible for a journal to claim that it is indexed in specific bibliographic databases. Authors should, however, double-check the claim's veracity before submitting it to the journal. We shall now skim through how to check a journal's indexing status in several databases recommended by the Board of Governors.

For Scopus:

1. Go to the site https://www.scopus.com/sources
2. Select "Title" or "ISSN" from the dropdown arrow type the title or ISSN accordingly and click on the "Find sources" button
3. From the search result, click on the target journal title
4. The indexed journal shows the "Scopus coverage years" (e.g. 2009 to 2019) and does not show "(coverage discontinued in Scopus)" below the years.

A list of a few Indian medical journals which are indexed in the SCOPUS is given in medical Table 17.1.

Table 17.1: List of few Indian medical journals indexed in SCOPUS

Name of the Journal	Name of the Publisher
Indian Journal of Medical Research	Indian Council of Medical Research
Indian Journal of Medical Research, Supplement	Indian Council of Medical Research
Current Science	Indian Academy of Sciences
Proceedings of the Indian National Science Academy	Indian National Science Academy
National Medical Journal of India	All India Institute of Medical Sciences
Indian Journal of Agricultural Sciences	Indian Journal of Fisheries for the Indian Council of Agricultural Research

Contd...

Table 17.1: List of few Indian medical journals indexed in SCOPUS

Name of the Journal	Name of the Publisher
Indian Journal of Physiology and Pharmacology	All India Institute of Medical Sciences
International Journal of Medical Toxicology and Legal Medicine	All India Institute of Medical Sciences
Advances in Dynamical Systems and Applications	Research India Publications
Indian Journal of Medical Research	Indian Council of Medical Research

For PubMed Central (PMC)

1. Visit https://www.ncbi.nlm.nih.gov/pmc/journals
2. Type the journal title in the search box given below "Search for journals" and click on the search button
3. On the search result page, the indexed journal shows "Full" in the "Participation level" column
4. You can also ensure that the latest volume is present in the PMC archive by clicking on the journal title hypertext

For MEDLINE

1. Visit https://www.ncbi.nlm.nih.gov/nlmcatalog
2. Type the journal title or ISSN in the search box and click on the search button
3. The journal details will be shown if it is in the National Library of Medicine (NLM) catalogue
4. Check the "Current indexing status." The indexed journal shows "Currently indexed for MEDLINE"

For EBSCO

1. Visit https://www.ebsco.com/title-lists
2. Look for the area of expertise you need like "Medicine" or "Dentistry"
3. Click on "Excel" or "HTML" that appears next to the coverage list
4. Check the indexing start date and stop date for the journal of interest
5. Make sure that the indexing stop date is empty otherwise, it means that the journal is not indexed in EBSCO anymore

For Clarivate Analytics (Previously known as Thomson Reuters/ISI)

1. Go to http://mjl.clarivate.com/
2. In the search field, write the full journal name.
3. In coverage, if you see Science Citation Index Expanded (SCIE), this means that the journal is indexed.
4. A lower level of indexing is Emerging Sources Citation Index (ESCI).

'H'-index

What does H-Index mean?

H-index also known as the Hirsch index was created by Jorge E. Hirsch in 2005 and is commonly referred to as the "h-index."

A scientist or scholar's productivity and the impact of their publications through citations are both intended to be gauged by the author-level indicator known as the h-index. A journal's or author's highest number of papers (h) with at least (h) number of citations are counted to determine the h-index. The h-index must rise to publish high-calibre studies. The researcher should make sure that they have not published any articles in publications that are predatory or false. The author should continuously publish new original research publications. Even though submitting more reviews might occasionally result in more citations, this eventually raises a profile's h-index. This index provides a precise snapshot of a person's research performance by capturing research output, i.e. it assesses the impact of an individual researcher.

Calculated by: Total number of publications of an author which has been cited by other authors at least the same number of times.

Example: When a researcher has authored 15 papers, and each of those papers has received a minimum of 15 citations, their h-index reaches a value of 15. This index is extremely helpful for comparing researchers with similar levels of experience. In gist, this index aids in comparing scholars who publish in the same journal categories and who work in fields, departments, or other comparable contexts, capturing a precise moment in time of a researcher's performance.

i10-index

A recent journal metric is the i10-index, which was introduced by Google Scholar in 2011. It is an easy-to-use indexing metric that may be discovered by counting the total number of papers published in a journal that has received at least 10 citations. i10-index also contributes to giving any student profile more weight. The i10-index's key benefit is its ease in calculating. Also, access to these measurements is simple and free, much thanks to Google Scholar.

A researcher who has received at least 10 citations for every 25 articles published has an i10-index of 25, which indicates that out of all publications. The i10-index varies depending on the researcher. It primarily depends on the research's topic and subfield.

Other indexes:

- m index
- g index
- w index

Suggested software to calculate the h-index:

- Scopus.
- Web of Science
- Google Scholar

What is a Journal Impact Factor?

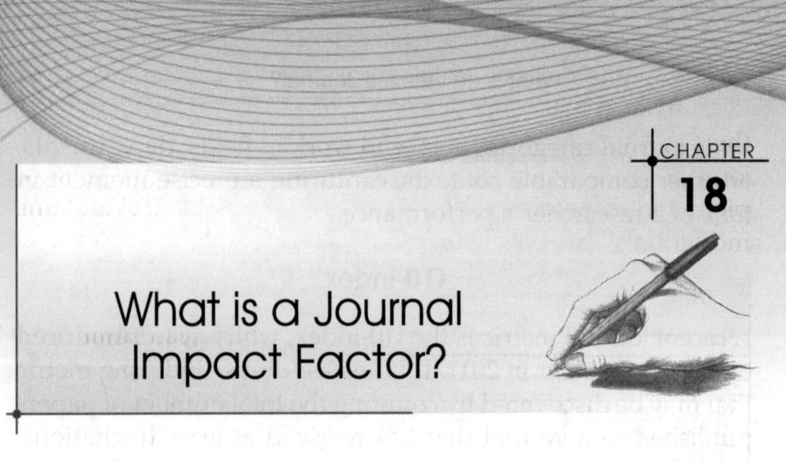

The Impact Factor (IF) is a commonly used indicator of a journal's relevance in its subject. Eugene Garfield, Founder of the Institute for Scientific Information, was the first to introduce this. Although IF is frequently used by institutions and clinicians, many people are unaware of the procedure for calculating the journal IF, its significance, and how it might be employed. The IF of a journal is a statistic that indicates the average number of citations to articles published in journals, books, theses, project reports, newspapers, and other types of publications. Table 18.1 contains the list of a few journals which have high IF.

The impact factor can only be calculated after a minimum of three years of publishing; hence, new journals' IF cannot be calculated. Over two years, the journal with the highest IF published the most frequently cited articles. Unlike the "H-index," the IF only pertains to journals, not individual publications, or scientists. "Citation impact" is a better term for the quantity of citations an individual publication receives. The IF of a journal in a particular year is the average number of citations received per article published in that journal during the previous two years. For example, if a journal's IF was three in 2008, each of its papers published in 2006 and 2007 received an average of three citations in 2008. The 2008 IFs were published in 2009, but they could not be calculated until the indexing agency had processed all the 2008 articles.

The determination of IF for the journal in which a person has written articles is a hotly debated topic. Nonetheless, because there is "a vast variety from article to paper within a single journal" and "in an ideal world, evaluators would read each piece and make personal assessments," "misuse in evaluating individuals" has been warned.

Table 18.1: List of a few medical journals with high impact factor

Name of the journal	Impact factor
CA—A Cancer Journal for Clinicians	223.679
New England Journal of Medicine	74.699
The Lancet	60.392
Nature Reviews Clinical Oncology	53.276
Nature Reviews Cancer	53.030
Nature Reviews Immunology	44.019
Nature	42.778
Nature Reviews Disease Primers	40.689
Cell	38.637
Nature Medicine	36.130
Nature Reviews Microbiology	34.209
The Lancet Infectious Diseases	24.446

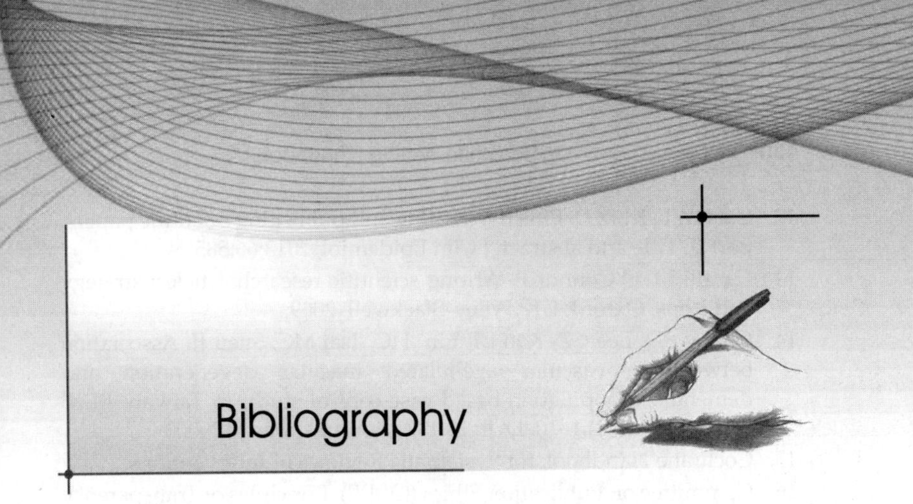

Bibliography

1. Acta Sci, Agron. How to write the discussion section of a scientific article, Vol. 41 Maringa 2019 Epub Mar 28, 2019.
2. Alexandrov AV, Hennerici MG. Writing good abstracts. Cerebrovasc Dis. 2007;23:256–9.
3. Annesley TM. The title says it all. Clin Chem. 2010;56:357–60.
4. Annesley TM. The discussion section: your closing argument. Clinical Chemistry, 2010;56(11):1671–4. DOI: 10.1373/clinchem.2010.155358
5. Anstey A. Writing style: Abstract thoughts. Br J Dermatol. 2014;171: 205–6.
6. Arma an A. How to write an introduction section of a scientific article? Turkish journal of urology, 2013;39(Suppl 1):8–9. https://doi.org/10.5152/tud.2013.046
7. Barbieri NL, Nielsen DW, Wannemuehler Y, Cavender T, Hussein A, Yan SG, Logue CM. mcr-1 identified in avian pathogenic Escherichia coli (APEC). PLoS ONE, 2017;12:1–13. DOI: 10.1371/journal.pone. 0172997
8. Blum A, Klueva N, Nguyen HT. Wheat cellular thermotolerance is related to yield under heat stress. Euphytica, 2001;117(2):117–23.
9. Boeck HD, Lemmens CMHM, Zavalloni C, Gielen B, Malchair S, Carnol M, Nijs I, et al. Biomass production in experimental grasslands of different species richness during three years of climate warming. Biogeosciences, 2008;5(2):585–94.
10. Bolnick DI. Snowberg LK, Hirsch PE, Lauber CL, Org E, Parks B, Svanbäck R. Individual diet has sex-dependent effects on vertebrate gut microbiota. Nature Communications, 2014;5(4500):1–13. DOI: 10.1038/ncomms5500
11. Brandi D Tuttle, Megan von Isenburg, Connie Schardt, and Anne Powers. PubMed instruction for medical students: searching for a better way. Medical reference services quarterly, 2009;28(3):199–210.

12. Cals JWL, Kotz D. Effective writing and publishing scientific papers, part II: Title and abstract. J Clin Epidemiol, 2013;66:585.

13. Cargill M, O'Connor P. Writing scientific research articles: strategy and steps. Oxford, UK: Wiley-Blackwell. 2009.

14. Chung SD, Lee CZ, Kao LT, Lin HC, Tsai MC, Sheu JJ. Association between neovascular age-related macular degeneration and dementia: a population-based case-control study in Taiwan. PLoS ONE, 2015;10(3):1–10. DOI: 10.1371/journal.pone.0120003

15. Cochrane Handbook for Systematic Reviews of Interventions.

16. Committee on Publication Ethics (COPE). Principles of Transparency and Best Practice in Scholarly Publishing, Version 2, 2015. Accessed on June 17, 2017.

17. Côté-Leclerc F, Duchesne GB, Bolduc P, Gélinas-Lafrenière A, Santerre C, Desrosiers J, Levasseur M. How does playing adapted sports affect the quality of life of people with mobility limitations? Results from a mixed-method sequential explanatory study. Health and Quality of Life Outcomes, 2017;15:1–8. DOI: 10.1186/s12955-017-0597-9

18. David Moher, Alessandro Liberati, Jennifer Tetzlaff, Douglas G Altman, Prisma Group, et al. Preferred reporting items for systematic reviews and meta-analyses: the PRISMA statement. PLoS med, 6(7):e1000097, 2009.

19. Day RA, Gastel B. How to write and publish a scientific paper. Westport, CT: Greenwood Press. 2006.

20. Deeks JJ, Higgins JPT, Altman DG (editors). Chapter 10: Analysing data and undertaking meta-analyses. In: Higgins JPT, Thomas J, Chandler J, Cumpston M, Li T, Page MJ, Welch VA (editors). Cochrane Handbook for Systematic Reviews of Interventions version 6.0 (updated July 2019). Cochrane, 2019.

21. DeMaria AN. How do I get a paper accepted? J Am Coll Cardiol. 2007; 49:1666–7.

22. Devi MJ, SinclairTR, Beebe SE, Rao IM. Comparison of common bean (Phaseolus vulgaris L.) genotypes for nitrogen fixation tolerance to soil drying. Plant and Soil, 2013;364(1–2):29–37. DOI: 10.1007/s11104-012-1330-4

23. Dimitriou M, Rallidis LS, Theodoraki EV, Kalafati IP, Kolovou G, Dedoussis GV. Exclusive olive oil consumption has a protective effect on coronary artery disease; overview of the THISEAS study. Public Health Nutrition, 2015;19(6):1081–1087. DOI: 10.1017/S1368980015002244

24. Docherty M, Smith R. The case for structuring the discussion of scientific papers: much the same as that for structuring abstracts.

British Medical Journal, 1999;318(7193):1224–5. DOI: 10.1136/bmj.318.7193.1224

25. Editorial, "Go forth and replicate!", Nature 536, 373 (2016). 4 Fang FC, Casadevall A. "Competitive Science: Is Competition Ruining Science?", Infection and Immunity 2015;83(4):1229.

26. Elsevier. Publishing Ethics Resource Kit (PERK). Available at: elsevier.com/editors/perk/plagiarism-complaints. Accessed on June 17, 2017.

27. Equator Network reporting guidelines.

28. Esposito M. The impact factor: It is use, misuse, and significance. Int J Prosthet Dent. 2011;24:85.

29. Everard A, Geurts L, Caesar R, Van Hul M, Matamoros S, Duparc T, Cani PD, et al. Intestinal epithelial MyD88 is a sensor switching host metabolism towards obesity according to nutritional status. Nature Communications, 2014;5(5648):1–12. DOI: 10.1038/ncomms6648

30. Falavigna A, De Faoite D, Blauth M, Kates SL. Basic steps to writing a paper: Practice makes perfect. The Bangkok Medical Journal, 2017;13(1):114–9.

31. Fassoulaki A, Papilas K, Paraskeva A, Patris K. Impact factor bias and proposed adjustments for it is determination. Acta Anaesthesiol Scand. 2002;46:902–5.

32. Feng J He, Graham A MacGregor. Effect of modest salt reduction on blood pressure: a meta-analysis of randomized trials. Implications for public health. Journal of human hypertension, 2002;16(11):761.

33. Foote M. The proof of the pudding: how to report results and write a good discussion. Chest, 2009;135(3):866–8. DOI: 10.1378/chest.08-2613

34. Frye MJ, Hough-Goldstein J. Plant architecture and growth response of kudzu (Fabales: Fabaceae) to simulated insect herbivory. Environmental Entomology, 2013;42(5):936–41.DOI:10.1603/EN12270.

35. Garfield E. The history and meaning of the journal impact factor. JAMA. 2006;295:90–3.

36. Glasman-Deal H. Science research writing for non-native speakers of English. London, UK: Imperial College Press, 2010.

37. Glass GV. Primary, Secondary and meta-analysis of research. Educ Researcher 1976;10:3–8.

38. Guilford WH. Teaching peer review and the process of scientific writing. Advances in Physiology Education 2001;25:167–75.

39. Harley CD, Hixon MA, Levin LA. Scientific Writing and Publishing Guide for Students. Bulletin of the Ecological Society of America, 2004;85:74–8.

40. Hess DR. How to write an effective discussion. Respiratory Care, 2004;49(10):1238–41.

41. Hiruma K, Gerlach N, Sacristán S, Nakano RT, Hacquard S, Kracher B, Schulze-Lefert P, et al. Root endophyte Colletotrichum tofieldiae confers plant fitness benefits that are phosphate status dependent. Cell, 2016;165(2):464–74.

42. Hofmann AH. Scientific writing and communication: papers, proposals, and presentations. New York, NY: Oxford University Press, 2014.

43. Https://guides.library.umass.edu/Research_Impact/Author_Level_ Metrics

44. Huang Y, Martin LM, Isbell FI, Wilsey BJ. Is community persistence related to diversity? A test with prairie species in a long-term experiment. Basic and Applied Ecology, 2013;14(3):199–207. DOI: 10.1016/j.baae.2013.01.007

45. Illari PM, Williamson J. What is a mechanism? Thinking about mechanisms across the sciences. European Journal for Philosophy of Science, 2012;2(2):119–35. DOI: 10.1007/s13194-011-0038-2

46. IOM Standards for Systematic Reviews

47. Joanna Briggs Institute (JBI) Reviewer's Manual for Scoping Reviews

48. Johansson H, Jones HJ, Foreman J, Hemsted JR, Stewart K, Grima R, Halliday KJ. Arabidopsis cell expansion is controlled by a photothermal switch. Nature Communications, 2014;5(4848):1–8. DOI: 10.1038/ncomms5848

49. John E Hunter, Frank L Schmidt. Fixed effects vs. random effects meta-analysis models: implications for cumulative research knowledge. International Journal of Selection and Assessment, 2000;8(4):275–92.

50. Kay Dickersin. The existence of publication bias and risk factors for It is occurrence. Jama, 1990;263(10):1385–9.

51. Kleijn D, Winfree R, Bartomeus I, Carvalheiro LG, Henry M, Isaacs R, Potts SG, et al. Delivery of crop pollination services is an insufficient argument for wild pollinator conservation. Nature Communications, 2015;6(7414):1–8. DOI: 10.1038/ncomms8414

52. Korkala EA, Hugg TT, Jaakkola JJK. Awareness of climate change and the dietary choices of young adults in Finland: A population-based cross-sectional study. PLoS ONE, 2014;9:1–9. DOI: 10. 1371/journal.pone.0097480

53. Kutman BY, Kutman UB, Cakmak I. Nickel-enriched seed and externally supplied nickel improve growth and alleviate foliar urea damage in soybeans. Plant and Soil, 2013;363(1–2):61–75. DOI: 10.1007/s11104-012-1284-6

54. Kysh Lynn. Difference between a systematic review and a literature review. 2013. [figshare]. Available at: http://dx.doi.org/10.6084/m9.figshare.766364

55. Lake L, Sadras V O. The critical period for yield determination in chickpeas (Cicer arietinum L.). Field Crops Research, 2014;168(11): 1–7. DOI: 10.1016/j.fcr.2014.08.003

56. Liberati A, Altman DG, Tetzlaff J, Mulrow C, Gotzsche PC, Ioannidis JPA, Clarke M, Devereaux PF, Kleijnen J, Moher D. The PRISMA statement for reporting systematic reviews and meta-analysis of studies that evaluate health care interventions: explanation and elaboration. PLoS Med. 2009;6(7):1–28.

57. Liu W, Qiao C, Yang S, Bai W, Liu L. Microbial carbon use efficiency and priming effect regulate soil carbon storage under nitrogen deposition by slowing soil organic matter decomposition. Geoderma, 2018;332(7438):37–44. DOI: 10.1016/j.geoderma.2018.07.008

58. Liu X, Zhang Y, Han W, Tang A, Shen J, Cui Z, Zhang F, et al. Enhanced nitrogen deposition over China. Nature, 2013;494:459–63. DOI: 10.1038/nature11917

59. Methodological Expectations for Cochrane Intervention Reviews (MECIR) Manual.

60. Michel LA. How to prepare a scientific surgical paper: a practical approach. Acta Chirurgica Belgica, 2012;112(4):323–39.

61. Moher D, Liberati A, Tetzlaff J, Altman DG, The PRISMA Group. Preferred Reporting Items for Systematic Reviews and Meta-Analyses: The PRISMA Statement, 2009. PLoS Med 6(7): e1000097. doi:10.1371/journal. pmed1000097

62. Mummey DL, Rillig MC. The invasive plant species Centaurea maculosa alters arbuscular mycorrhizal fungal communities in the field. Plant and Soil, 2006;288(1):81–90. DOI: 10.1007/s11104-006-9091-6

63. Nakayama Y, Moriya T, Sakai F, Ikeda N, Shiozaki T, Hosoya T, Miyazaki T, et al. Oral administration of Lactobacillus gasseri SBT2055 is effective for preventing influenza in mice. Scientific Reports, 2014;4(4638):1–5. DOI: 10.1038/srep04638

64. Oaks JL, Gilbert M, Virani MZ, Watson RT, Meteyer CU, Rideout BC, Khan AA, et al. Diclofenac residues as the cause of vulture population decline in Pakistan. Nature, 2004;427(12):630–3. DOI: 10.1038/nature02317

65. Paez-Valencia J, Sanchez-Lares J, Marsh E, Dorneles LT, Santos MP, Sanchez D, Gaxiola RA, et al. Enhanced proton translocating pyrophosphatase activity improves nitrogen use efficiency in romaine lettuce. Plant Physiology, 2013;161(3):1557–69. DOI: 10.1104/pp.112.212852

66. Papanas N, Georgiadis GS, Maltezos E, Lazarides MK. Writing a research abstract: Eloquence in miniature. Int Angiol. 2012;31: 297–302.

67. PRISMA Statement on Systematic Review Reporting,2020 (http:// prisma-statement.org/)

68. Merton RK, The Sociology of Science: Theoretical and Empirical Investigations, University of Chicago Press, Chicago, IL, 1973.

69. Sue Duval and Richard Tweedie. Trim and fill: a simple funnel-plot–based method of testing and adjusting for publication bias in meta-analysis. Biometrics, 2000;56(2):455–63.

70. Kuhn TS. The Structure of Scientific Revolutions, 3rd ed., University of Chicago Press, Chicago, IL, 1996.

71. Takatani S, Hirayama T, Hashimoto T, Takahashi T, Motose H. Abscisic acid induces ectopic outgrowth in epidermal cells through cortical microtubule reorganization in Arabidopsis thaliana. Scientific Reports, 2015;5(11364):1–12. DOI: 10.1038/srep11364

72. Tan K, Chen W, Dong S, Liu X, Wang Y, Nieh JC. A neonicotinoid impairs olfactory learning in Asian honey bees (Apis cerana) exposed as larvae or as adults. Scientific Reports, 2015;5:1–8. DOI: 10.1038/srep10989

73. Tullu MS, Karande S. Writing a model research paper: A roadmap. J Postgrad Med. 2017;63:143–6.

74. University Grants Commission (UGC) Regulations (Promotion of Academic Integrity and Prevention of Plagiarism in Higher Education Institutions), 2018.

75. Van Zutphen M, Winkels RM, van Duijnhoven FJB, van Harten-GerrIt isen SA, Kok DEG, van Duijvendijk P, Kampman E, et al. An increase in physical activity after colorectal cancer surgery is associated with improved recovery of physical functioning: a prospective cohort study. BMC Cancer, 2017;17(1):1–9. DOI: 10.1186/s12885-017-3066-2

76. Vernon Booth: Writing a scientific paper. Biochem Soc. 1975;3:1–26.

77. Vic Hasselblad and Larry V Hedges. Meta-analysis of screening and diagnostic tests. Psychological Bulletin, 1995;117(1):167.

78. Wallwork, A. English for writing research papers. New York, NY: Springer, 2016.

79. Wiley.com: How to write a scientific abstract?

80. Yuan Z, Li L, Han X, Huang J, Jiang G, Wan S. Soil characteristics and nitrogen resorption in Stipa krylovii native to northern China. Plant and Soil, 2005;273(1):257–68. DOI: 10.1007/s11104-004-7941-7.

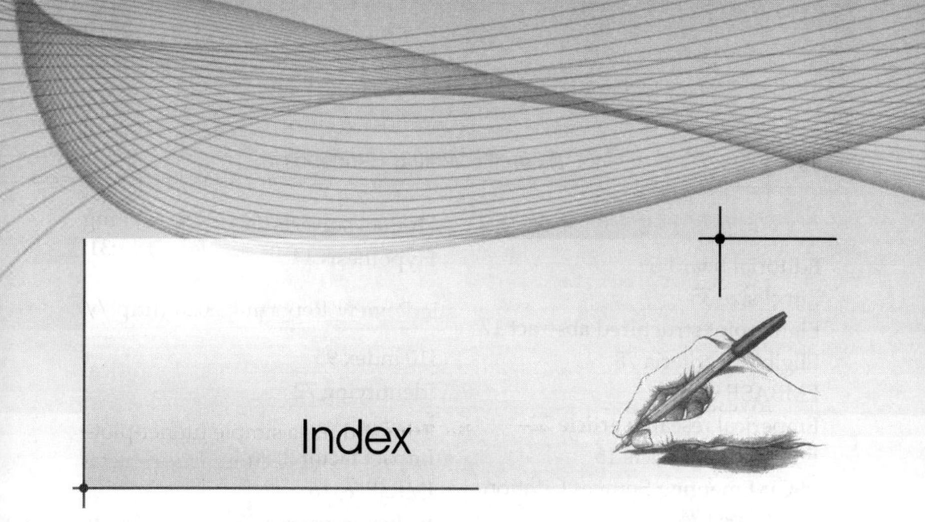

Index